ANATOMY AND
EMBRYOLOGY
OF THE HEAD
AND NECK

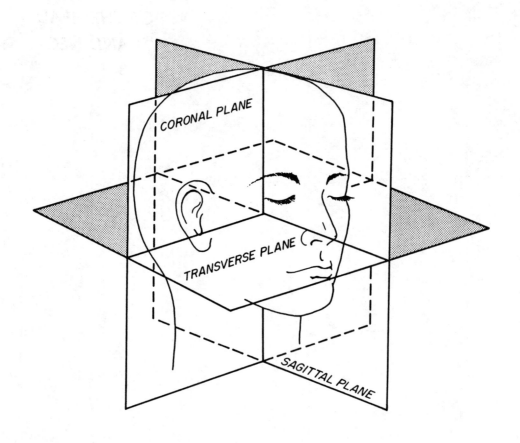

ANATOMY AND EMBRYOLOGY OF THE HEAD AND NECK

Holliston L. Riviere, Ph.D.

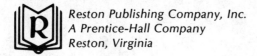
Reston Publishing Company, Inc.
A Prentice-Hall Company
Reston, Virginia

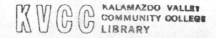

Library of Congress Cataloging in Publication Data

Riviere, Holliston L.
  Anatomy and embryology of the head and neck.

  Includes bibliographical references and index.
  1. Head.   2. Neck.   3. Embryology, Human.   I. Title.
[DNLM: 1. Head—Anatomy and histology.   2. Head—
Embryology.   3. Neck—Anatomy and histology.   4. Neck—
Embryology.   WE 705 R625a]
QM535.R58   611'.91   82-5215
ISBN 0-8359-0211-0   AACR2

© 1983 by
Reston Publishing Company, Inc.
Reston, Virginia 22090

10 9 8 7 6 5 4 3 2 1

Printed in the United States of America.

CONTENTS

PREFACE

This text is intended for use both as a primary text and as a review. To that end it is concise, presenting basic material in a manner that should be easy to assimilate. The student should have access to skeletal material and a good atlas of human anatomy. The learning objectives at the beginning of each chapter are intended to help the instructor and student decide upon the depth of study. The summaries at the end of most chapters make it easier for the student to review what he has just read and what types of information coincide with the depth of study he wishes to engage in. The study exercises are designed to help the student review material and test his knowledge. Some exercises have the simple objective of making the study of anatomy a more human task. Objectives, summaries, and exercises in italics are intended for more in-depth study.

Since I find my students copying figures and handouts and removing the labels for the purpose of study, I thought it might be helpful if some of the figures in this text appeared in an appendix without labels so that the student could test himself more easily. A piece of plastic overlay can be used over the figures so that they may be reused. They can also be used for quick quizzes in the classroom.

It is my sincere hope that the study aids included here make the study of anatomy an easier, more interesting, adventure. There really are few things more fascinating than the remarkable animal called man.

HLR

ACKNOWLEDGMENTS

The substance of this text is information acquired from many sources. Published sources are listed in the general reference section. But the contributions and support of former instructors, advisors, colleagues, students, and family are impossible to reference. I wish to acknowledge and thank them all. I also wish to thank Sharon Heller, who typed the manuscript, and Karen Christenson, who did the artwork.

*ANATOMY AND
EMBRYOLOGY
OF THE HEAD
AND NECK*

1

REVIEW
OF TERMS
AND CONCEPTS

LEARNING OBJECTIVES

At the conclusion of this chapter, the student should be able to:

1. Describe the three major planes of section.
2. Define the terms that describe relative position of structures.
3. Define the terms that describe movements associated with the head and neck.
4. *Describe the anatomic position.*

Before beginning to study the anatomy of the head and neck, it is necessary to define terms of anatomic reference. Since this text deals only with the anatomy of the head and neck, only terms relevant to these structures will be defined.

PLANES

All descriptions of anatomic relationships are based on a standard position of the body called the anatomic position. A person is in the anatomic position when he stands erect with his feet together and his arms at his sides with the palms of the hands forward. In the anatomic position, a vertical plane through the center of the body that divides it into right and left halves is called the median sagittal plane (Figure 1-1). All other planes parallel to the median sagittal plane are simply called sagittal planes. A vertical plane through the body at right angles to the median sagittal plane is called a coronal plane. A horizontal plane through the body at right angles to both the coronal and sagittal planes, producing a cross-section, is called a transverse or horizontal plane.

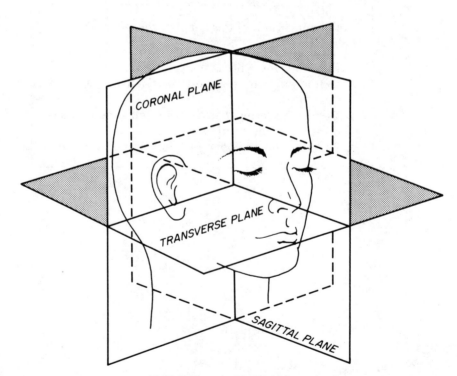

FIGURE 1-1   Planes of section.

POSITIONS

The ventral body surface is the front of the body. The dorsal body surface is the back of the body. The term *anterior* is sometimes used instead of ventral and *posterior* instead of dorsal.

Medial and *lateral* describe location relative to the median sagittal plane. The eyes are lateral to the nose but medial to the ears.

Superior and *inferior* refer to relative location in a vertical plane. The eyes are superior to the chin.

Proximal and *distal* refer to the relative distance of one structure from another. Proximal means closer and distal means further away from. The hand is distal to the shoulder.

Ipsilateral refers to the same side of the body, while *contralateral* refers to opposite sides. The right eye and ear are ipsilateral. The right eye is contralateral to the left ear.

Superficial and *deep* describe relative distance from a body surface. *Internal* and *external* describe relative distance from the center of a body structure or cavity.

MOVEMENTS

A wide range of movement of the head and cervical spine is possible. The head may be rotated to the left or right. The head and cervical spine may be flexed, bent forward, extended, or bent backward. The spinal column and head can also be flexed laterally as when the ear is moved toward the ipsilateral shoulder.

Protraction (or protrusion) is movement forward, while retraction (or retrusion) is movement backward as in movements of the jaw at the temporomandibular joint (TMJ). The tongue can also be protracted and retracted.

Two other terms used to describe the movement of the jaw are *elevation* and *depression*. To elevate the jaw is to close it and to depress the jaw is to open it.

CHAPTER SUMMARY

Plane of Section	Definition
Mid-sagittal	A vertical plane through the center of the body dividing it into right and left sides.
Sagittal	A vertical plane through the body parallel to the median sagittal plane.
Transverse	A horizontal plane at right angles to the sagittal and coronal planes which results in a cross-section.
Coronal	A vertical plane through the body at right angles to the sagittal plane. A mid-coronal plane would divide the body into front and back halves.

Relative position	Definition
Ventral	Front of the body
Dorsal	Back of the body
Medial	Toward the middle or mid-sagittal plane
Lateral	Toward the side or away from the mid-sagittal plane
Superior	Above, more toward the head
Inferior	Below, more toward the feet
Proximal	Closer to
Distal	Farther from
Ipsilateral	On the same side of the body
Contralateral	On opposite sides of the body
Superficial	Nearer the body surface
Deep	Farther from the body surface
Internal	Nearer the center of the body
External	Farther from the center of the body or nearer the surface
Rotation	Turning to the right or left, or in a circular pattern
Flexion	Bending the head forward (Bending the head laterally is also called lateral flexion.)
Extension	Bending the head backward
Protraction (Protrusion)	Projecting the jaw or tongue forward
Retraction (Retrusion)	Withdrawing the jaw or tongue
Elevation	Closing the jaw
Depression	Opening the jaw

STUDY EXERCISES

1. Describe the effect upon the body of a section in each of the following planes:

    A. Mid-sagittal
    B. Mid-coronal
    C. Transverse

2. Define each of the following terms, and state the term which is its opposite:

    A. Dorsal
    B. Distal
    C. Ipsilateral
    D. Medial
    E. Deep
    F. Inferior
    G. External

3. Using a mirror, observe the range of movement of the head and neck, jaw and tongue. Compare your mobility with that of one or more of your classmates.

4. *Why is it important to know the plane of section of anatomic material or drawings of such material?*

5. *Why is it important to be able to describe a structure in anatomic terms (ie., dorsal, superior, etc.)?*

2

THE
SKELETAL
SYSTEM

LEARNING OBJECTIVES

At the conclusion of this chapter, the student should be able to:

1. Describe the types of joints in the head and neck.
2. Recognize the typical cervical vertebrae, the atlas, and axis. *Identify the parts of these vertebrae and how they differ from one another.*
3. Identify the bones of the skull, their locations, surface features, processes, and foramina.
4. *Define the limits of the various fossae of the skull.*
5. *Name the major sutures and the bones that form them.*

THE JOINTS

A joint is a place where bones come together. There are two basic kinds of joints: those with little or no movement, and those which provide for free movement. Joints where little or no movement takes place are further divided into fibrous and cartilaginous types. Bones involved in fibrous joints are held together by specialized connective tissue fibers called collagen. The collagen fibers bridge the gap between the bones in an organized manner. The amount of movement in the joint depends upon the distance between the bones. The joints between most of the bones of the skull are a type of fibrous joint called a suture. Sutures are very wide and movable at birth but become increasingly smaller and tighter with age. They will be completely replaced by bone to form an immovable bony union in old age. Other fibrous joints in the head include the groove-type joint of the vomer and ethmoid bones, called schindylesis, and the joints between the teeth and their bony sockets called gomphoses (singular, gomphosis).

At a cartilaginous joint, the bones are joined by some type of cartilage. The joints between the bodies of the vertebrae are examples of this type. The bodies of the vertebrae are joined by fibrocartilage. The amount of movement depends upon the physical properties of the fibrocartilage.

Freely movable joints are called synovial joints. The bony ends, which are united at a synovial joint, are covered with a smooth layer of hyaline cartilage. The union is maintained by muscles and ligaments. A fibrous capsule surrounds the cartilage-covered ends of the bones and the space between the bones, and the capsule is lubricated by a liquid called synovial fluid. Sometimes a disc of fibrocartilage is suspended between the ends of the bones within the joint capsule. The amount and direction of movements depend upon the muscular and ligamentous attachments and the shape of the bones involved. The craniovertebral joints—joints between articular facets on vertebrae and temporomandibular joints—are examples of synovial joints in the head and neck.

THE CERVICAL SPINE

Seven cervical vertebrae comprise the cervical vertebral column. The first, second, and seventh vertebrae are atypical and will be described separately.

The typical cervical vertebrae is illustrated in Figure 2–1. It is composed of an anterior body and a posterior arch, which forms the vertebral foramen in which lies the spinal cord. The large body faces

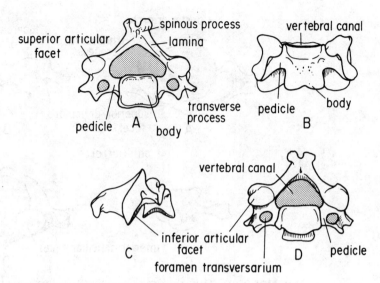

FIGURE 2–1 Typical cervical vertebrae: (A) superior view, (B) anterior view, (C) lateral view, (D) inferior view.

anteriorly and is joined with the vertebrae above and below by intervertebral discs. Bilateral transverse processes extend laterally from the body. The foramen transversarium, located in each transverse process, transmits the vertebral artery.

The vertebral arch is formed by the pedicles and the laminae. The pedicles are short, thick, bony projections from the posterior surface of the body of the vertebrae. Each pedicle is notched above and below. When the vertebrae are articulated, opposing notches of two vertebrae form the intervertebral foramen, from which the spinal nerves emerge. The laminae are flat projections from the pedicles. They meet posteriorly, completing the arch. The spinous process arises from the junction of the laminae and projects downward and backward. The spinous processes of cervical vertebrae are bifid.

Four articular facets, two superior and two inferior, are located at the junctions of the pedicles and the laminae. They form joints with the appropriate facets of vertebrae immediately above and below.

The first cervical vertebra is called the atlas (Figure 2–2). It articulates superiorly with the skull and is very different from the typical vertebrae just described. The atlas has no body. It consists of anterior and posterior arches and two lateral masses. During development, the body of the atlas fuses with that of the second cervical vertebra, the axis, to form a bony projection called the dens. On the inner surface of the anterior arch is a small facet for articulation with the

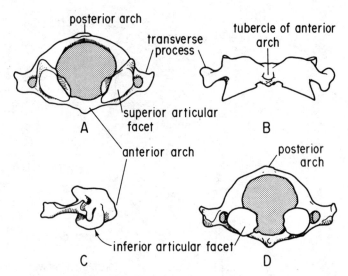

FIGURE 2–2   The atlas: (A) superior view, (B) anterior view, (C) lateral view, (D) inferior view.

dens. The lateral masses connect the anterior arch with the posterior arch. The masses bear superior and inferior articular facets for atlanto-occipital and atlanto-axial joints respectively. A small, roughened area on the inside of the anterior end of each lateral mass serves for attachment of the transverse ligament of the atlas. This ligament holds the dens in place against the articular facet. A transverse process projects laterally from each lateral mass, and each contains a foramen transversarium. The posterior arch completes the vertebral foramen. A small posterior tubercle at the center of the posterior arch represents the spinous process.

The second cervical vertebra, or axis, is also modified but not as much as the atlas (Figure 2–3). The dens projects from the superior aspect of the body of the axis. The dens has an articular facet on its anterior surface, and its posterior surface is grooved for the transverse ligament of the atlas. The dens is flanked on either side by large surfaces for articulation with the atlas above. The inferior articular facets are located on the inferior surface. The pedicles and laminae complete the posterior vertebral arch. A bifid spinous process projects from the posterior junction of the laminae.

The seventh cervical vertebra has some of the characteristics of the thoracic vertebrae. The spinous process is not bifid and is visible superficially as a bump at the base of the neck. It is sometimes called the vertebra prominens.

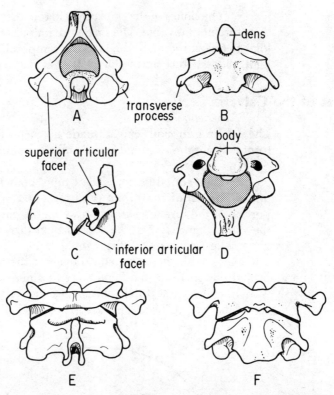

FIGURE 2–3   **The axis: (A) superior view, (B) anterior view, (C) lateral view, (D) inferior view, (E) posterior view of articulated atlas and axis, (F) anterior view of articulated atlas and axis.**

Movement at the atlanto-occipital joint is limited by the shape of the articular facets and the ligaments and joint capsules to an anterior and posterior rock (nodding) motion. Rotation of the head occurs at the atlanto-axial joint and is limited again by the joint capsules and ligaments.

THE SKULL

The skull may be divided into two parts: that portion which houses the brain, the cranium, and the remainder, which forms the skeleton of the face. The cranium may be further divided. The roof is called the calvaria, and the floor is called the cranial base. Many bones contribute to both the facial skeleton and the brain case. These divisions are used for the sake of convenience rather than anatomic accuracy.

The bones of the skull are held together by suture joints and are therefore not movable. The single exception is the temporomandibular joint between the mandible and the temporal bone. This is a synovial joint, the structure and movement of which will be discussed.

Bones of the Calvaria

The calvaria, or skull cap, is made up of portions of four bones: the frontal bone, the occipital bone, and the paired parietal bones.

The Frontal Bone.   The frontal bone forms the forehead and upper portion of the orbits (Figure 2–4). The large, flat, squamous portion of the forehead articulates with the parietal bones at the top of the skull (Figure 2–5). The supraorbital margins end laterally on the zygomatic processes of the frontal bone. This short, thick process articulates with the zygomatic bone. At the medial one-third of the orbital margins is a small notch (or foramen), the supraorbital notch. Above each supraorbital margin is a curved prominence called the superciliary arch. The arches are joined medially by a flat elevation, the

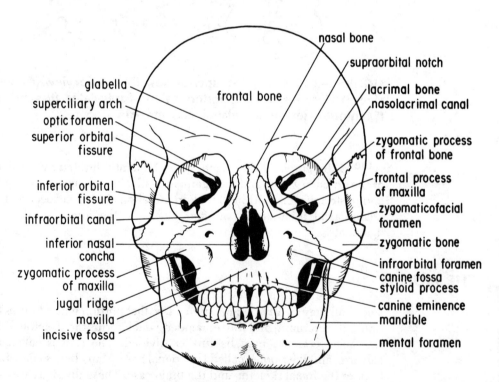

FIGURE 2–4   Frontal aspect of the skull.

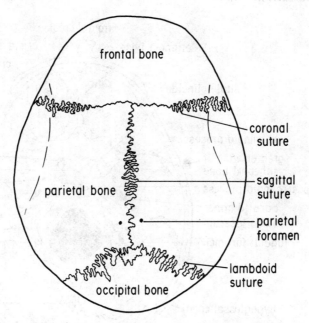

FIGURE 2-5   Superior aspect of the calvaria.

glabella. Below the glabella is the nasal portion of the frontal bone. The small nasal bones, the maxillae (singular-maxilla), and the ethmoid bones articulate here. The nasal spine of the frontal bone projects from the midline of the nasal area and forms a small part of the nasal septum. This spine is partially hidden by the nasal bones. If the frontal bone is disarticulated and the orbital surface viewed, small, bony pockets can be seen on each side in the orbital wall. These are the roofs of the ethmoid air cells of the ethmoid bone. They are a part of the system of nasal sinuses. The frontal sinuses are connected to the most anterior of the air cells and are located in the frontal bone behind the superciliary arches.

The intracranial surface of the frontal bone supports and protects the frontal portion of the brain. Unlike the smooth intraorbital surface, the surface in the cranium is ridged and grooved like the brain it supports. At the midline of the squamous portion is a ridge, the frontal crest, which serves for attachment of the *dura* (Figure 2-6).

The Parietal Bones. The paired parietal bones form the middle of the roof of the cranium (Figures 2-5 and 2-7). Their junction at the midline of the calvaria is called the sagittal suture. They are rectangular, broad, and curved. Each parietal bone articulates anteriorly with the squamous part of the frontal bone. The resulting

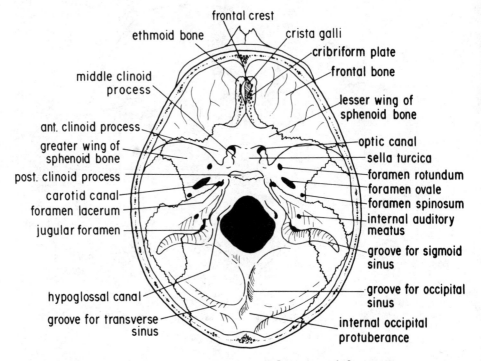

FIGURE 2-6   Intracranial aspect of the skull.

suture is called the coronal suture. Inferiorly, the parietal meets the temporal bone, and posteriorly it meets the occipital bone. The outer lateral surface of each parietal is marked by two curving lines, the superior and inferior temporal lines. These lines mark the attachment of the temporal fascia and temporalis muscle respectively. Sometimes a small parietal foramen is located in each bone near the posterior end of the sagittal suture.

The intracranial surface of the parietal is etched by a network of grooves for the middle meningeal artery (Figure 2-8). A deep groove follows the internal line of the sagittal suture. This groove houses a venous sinus, the superior sagittal sinus.

The Occipital Bone. The occipital bone completes the posterior portion of the skull (Figures 2-6, 2-9, and 2-10). It consists of a squamous portion, two lateral or condylar portions, and a basilar portion. The basilar and condylar portions form the floor of the posterior cranial base. They surround a large opening, the foramen magnum, through which the spinal cord exits the cranial cavity. The squamous portion curves upward to meet the posterior margin of the parietal bones, thereby completing the calvaria. The junction between the occipital and parietal bones is the lambdoid suture.

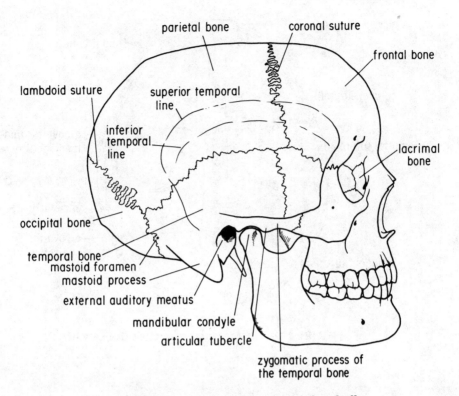

FIGURE 2–7 Lateral aspect of the skull.

    The external surface of the squamous portion of the occipital bone is marked by several ridges or lines for muscle attachment (Figure 2–9). Near the base of the squama at the midline is a prominence called the external occipital protuberance. Slightly above and curving laterally from the protuberance is the supreme nuchal line. Slightly below the supreme line, the superior nuchal line follows a similar course. The inferior nuchal line is a more prominent transverse ridge at the base of the squama. These lines mark the attachments of the posterior neck muscles.

    The internal surface of the squama of the occipital bone is divided into four depressions or fossae by prominent vertical and transverse grooves. The two superior fossae house the occipital lobes of the cerebral hemispheres of the brain. The inferior fossae house the two lobes of the cerebellum. The point where the grooves cross is the internal occipital protuberance. The grooves house dural venous sinuses, which will be described with the venous system.

    On the external surface of the condylar portion of the occipital bone, the occipital condyles flank the foramen magnum (Figure 2–10).

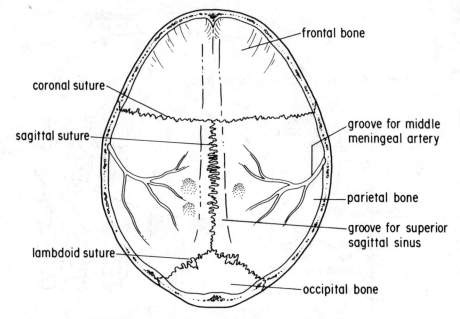

FIGURE 2–8   Intracranial aspect of the calvaria.

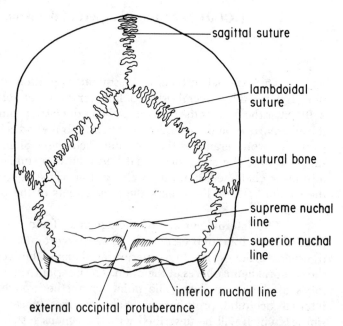

FIGURE 2–9   Posterior aspect of the skull.

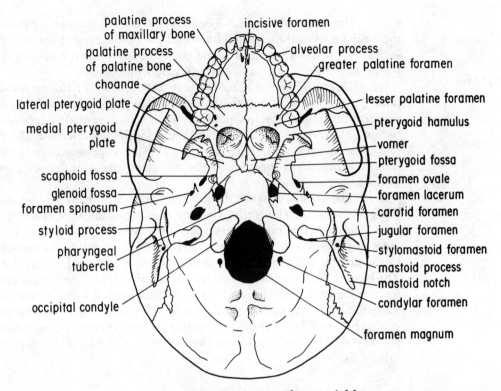

palatine process
of maxillary bone

incisive foramen

palatine process
of palatine bone

alveolar process

greater palatine foramen

choanae

lateral pterygoid plate

lesser palatine foramen

medial pterygoid
plate

pterygoid hamulus

vomer

pterygoid fossa

scaphoid fossa

foramen ovale

glenoid fossa

foramen lacerum

foramen spinosum

carotid foramen

styloid process

jugular foramen

stylomastoid foramen

pharyngeal
tubercle

mastoid process

mastoid notch

occipital condyle

condylar foramen

foramen magnum

FIGURE 2–10   The cranial base.

The condyles articulate with the atlas. On the medial surface of each
condyle, almost within the foramen magnum, is the hypoglossal canal
for transmission of the hypoglossal nerve. Behind each condyle is a
small depression, the condylar fossa. The condylar foramen may be
found in the floor of the fossa, but this is variable.

The basilar portion of the occipital bone is a short, rectangular
projection of bone from the anterior lip of the foramen magnum
forward. It articulates with the sphenoid bone. The internal surface is
smooth and supports the brain stem. The external surface is roughened.
A small projection, the pharyngeal tubercle, serves as attachment for the
fascia of the pharynx.

Bones of the Cranial Base

The bones of the cranial base are the sphenoid temporal and basilar
portion of the occipital bone already described. Along with the bones of
the calvaria, they complete the brain case.

The Sphenoid Bone.   The sphenoid bone is situated between the basilar part of the occipital bone and the frontal bone (Figures 2–6 and 2–11). It has a complex shape consisting of a body, two greater wings, two lesser wings, and two pterygoid processes.

The body of the sphenoid bone articulates with the occipital bone posteriorly and the ethmoid and vomer bones anteriorly. It is square and contains the sphenoid sinuses. The intracranial surface has two sets of processes, the middle and posterior clinoid processes. These mark the anterior and posterior margins of a depression, the sella turcica. In life, the hypophysis, or pituitary gland, sits in the deepest part of the sella turcica.

The greater wings of the sphenoid project from the sides of the body like wings of a butterfly. They are concave on the intracranial surface. The posterior margins articulate with the temporal bones. The anterior portions form the postero-lateral wall of the orbit. The portion of the greater wing that can be seen in the orbit is roughly triangular. The base of the triangle is toward the lateral orbital rim. The apex points toward the back of the orbit. One side of the triangle forms the inferior margin of a slit-like opening in the back of the orbit called the superior orbital fissure. The other side of the triangle forms the lateral margin of another slit-like opening in the floor of the orbit called the inferior orbital fissure.

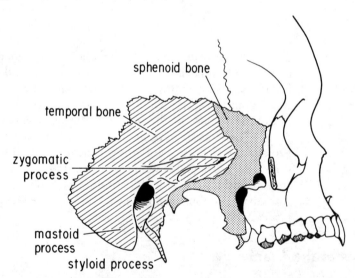

FIGURE 2–11   Diagram of the extent of the temporal bone (lined) and the sphenoid bone (stippled) on the lateral aspect of the skull.

Three foramina pierce the greater wings of the sphenoid on its intracranial aspect. The foramen rotundum is located just behind the medial end of the superior orbital fissure. It transmits the maxillary division of the trigeminal nerve. Behind this foramen and slightly lateral is the larger foramen ovale, which transmits the mandibular division of the trigeminal nerve. Posterior and lateral to the foramen ovale is the foramen spinosum. The middle meningeal artery enters the cranial cavity via the foramen spinosum. The foramen is so named because it is located at the base of the sphenoid spine on the extracranial aspect.

The lesser wings of the sphenoid project from the upper anterior aspect of the body. They articulate with the posterior margins of the frontal bone and the ethmoid. They form the upper posterior portion of the orbit and the superior boundary of the superior orbital fissure. At the origin of each lesser wing, the anterior clinoid process projects backward along the lateral edge of the sella turcica. The foramen hidden underneath the lesser wing between the anterior clinoid process and the body of the sphenoid is the optic canal. The groove for the optic chiasma lies between the two optic canals across the anterior margin of the sella turcica. The optic nerves exit the orbit through the optic canals.

The pterygoid processes descend from the extracranial surface of the sphenoid bone at the junctions of the greater wing and body (Figure 2-10). The processes flank the posterior nasal openings or choanae. Each process consists of a medial and lateral plate. The fossa between the plates is the pterygoid fossa. A small depression at the base of each medial plate is the scaphoid fossa. A small hook-like process, the pterygoid hamulus, curves laterally from the free end of each medial plate.

The Temporal Bone.   The temporal bone is a very complex and important member of the cranial base (Figures 2-6, 2-7, 2-10, 2-11, and 2-12). It consists of a flat, squamous part, which completes the cranial vault; petro-mastoid and tympanic parts, which house the ear; and the styloid process.

The squama articulates with the sphenoid bone in front and below and the parietal bone above. The inner surface is grooved by branches of the middle meningeal artery. The long, slender zygomatic process of the temporal bone projects anteriorly from the base of the outer surface of the squamous portion (Figure 2-11).

The depression on the undersurface of the temporal bone just medial to the origin of the zygomatic process is the glenoid or mandibular fossa. The mandibular articulation, or temporomandibular joint, is located here. The fossa is bounded anteriorly by a ridge, the

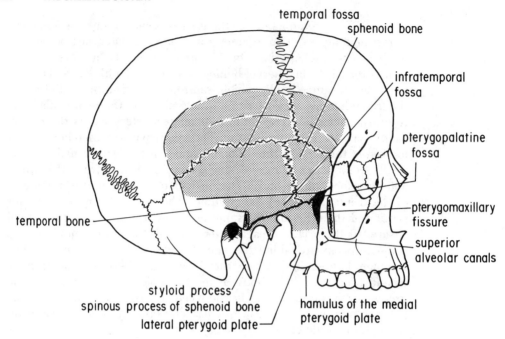

temporal fossa
sphenoid bone
infratemporal fossa
pterygopalatine fossa
pterygomaxillary fissure
superior alveolar canals
temporal bone
styloid process
spinous process of sphenoid bone
lateral pterygoid plate
hamulus of the medial pterygoid plate

FIGURE 2–12   Lateral aspect of the skull showing the extent of the temporal fossa (stippled area).

articular tubercle. The glenoid fossa abuts against the lateral end of the tympanic portion of the temporal bone.

Laterally, a large opening, the external auditory meatus, can be seen. Posterior to the meatus, the conical mastoid process projects downward. The mastoid portion of the temporal bone articulates with the occipital bone posteriorly and inferiorly, and the parietal bone superiorly. The mastoid foramen is located behind the mastoid process near the lambdoid suture. The mastoid process is a honeycomb of air cells that communicate with the middle ear in the petrous portion of the temporal bone. The mastoid notch grooves the undersurface of the process. A small foramen, the stylomastoid foramen, is located near the anterior end of the groove. This foramen transmits the facial nerve. The styloid process is a narrow, pointed spicule of bone that arises immediately anterior to the stylomastoid foramen.

The word *petrous* means rock-like, and indeed this portion of the temporal bone is very hard. It houses the ear. From the intracranial aspect, the petrous portion is a wedge of bone. It has a base, an anterior surface and a posterior surface. The anterior surface bulges slightly near its lateral end. This bulge, the arcuate eminence, covers one of the semicircular canals of the inner ear. At the medial end of the anterior surface is a slight depression for the trigeminal or semilunar ganglion. A large, jagged foramen at the medial end of the anterior surface of the petrous part is the foramen lacerum.

The posterior surface of the petrous part of the temporal bone slopes back toward the occipital bone. A foramen, the internal auditory meatus, is located at the medial one third of this side. Directly below the internal meatus is the jugular foramen where the jugular vein originates. A deep "S"-shaped groove sweeps laterally from the jugular foramen and is continuous with the transverse grooves of the occipital bone previously described. The "S"-shaped depression is the groove for the sigmoid venous sinus.

The base of the petrous portion of the temporal bone is viewed from the inferior aspect of the skull. From this view, the jugular foramina can be seen just lateral to the anterior margin of the occipital condyles. Immediately in front of the jugular foramen is the entrance to the carotid canal. The carotid canal is a short tube of bone that transmits the internal carotid artery into the cranial cavity. From the inferior aspect, the petrous and auditory portions of the temporal bone appear to be separated from surrounding bone by deep fissures. Posteriorly, a jagged crack runs forward from the jugular foramen to the anterior end of the carotid canal. In life, this fissure is filled with cartilage. Cartilage also completes the carotid canal filling in the extracranial opening of the foramen lacerum. Therefore, no structure traverses the foramen lacerum. The foramen does not exist in the living subject. It is created by the removal or deterioration of cartilage.

The Eustachian tube from the middle ear emerges from the ear in a fissure just posterior to the foramen spinosum. The tube is cartilaginous from that point to the pharyngeal opening near the base of the pterygoid process.

Bones of the Facial Skeleton

The bones of the facial skeleton are the ethmoid, vomer, palatine, nasal, inferior nasal concha, lacrimal, maxillary, zygomatic, and mandible. The first six are associated with the nose and/or orbits. The maxillary bones, zygomatic bones, and mandible complete the skeleton of the face.

The Ethmoid Bone.   The ethmoid bone forms the roof of the nasal cavity, part of the nasal septum, and a portion of the medial wall of the orbit (Figures 2–8, 2–13, and 2–14). It consists of the cribriform plate, a perpendicular plate, and two lateral labyrinths.

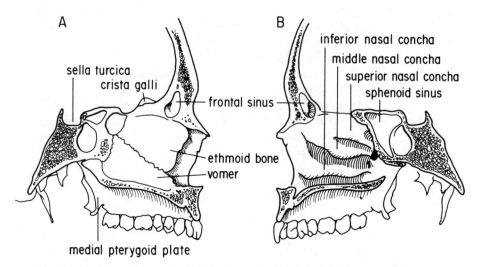

FIGURE 2–13 Bony nasal septum and cavity: (A) sagittal section showing the bony nasal septum, (B) nasal cavity with nasal septum removed.

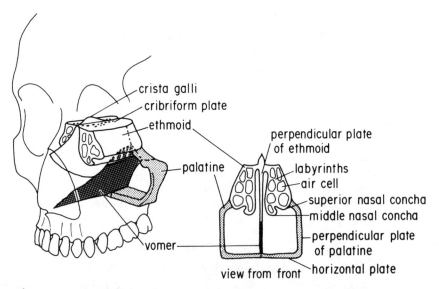

Figure 2–14 Relationship of the ethmoid, palatine, and vomer bones.

The cribriform plate can be seen in the cranial cavity above the nasal cavities and between the orbital plates of the frontal bone. It is perforated for transmission of the olfactory nerves. A sharp process, the crista galli, projects upward in the median plane. The perpendicular plate projects downward from the center of the undersurface of the cribriform plate into the nasal cavity, partially dividing the cavity into right and left sides. The plate forms the upper portion of the bony nasal septum. The labyrinths are two roughly cuboidal pieces of bone on either side of the perpendicular plate. Each consists of thin-walled groups of air cells sandwiched between two vertical plates of bone. The ethmoid bone is situated so that the inner or medial bony plate forms the lateral nasal wall. Two processes, the superior and middle nasal conchae, project from this surface into the nasal cavity. The lateral side of each labyrinth or orbital plate forms part of the medial wall of the corresponding orbit. Like the other paranasal sinuses, the ethmoid air cells communicate with the nasal cavity.

The Vomer.   The vomer is a thin plate of bone that forms the inferior portion of the bony nasal septum (Figures 2-13 and 2-14). It articulates above with the perpendicular plate of the ethmoid bone and below with the midline of the floor of the nasal cavities. The vomer articulates with the body of the sphenoid bone behind the nasal cavities.

The Palatine Bone.   The paired palatine bones form the posterior one-fourth of the hard palate and the posterolateral wall of the nasal cavities and a small portion of the posterior floor of the orbit (Figures 2-10 and 2-14). Each bone consists of a horizontal and a perpendicular plate. The horizontal plates form the remainder of the hard palate and articulate with the palatal processes of the maxillae in front and each other at the midline. The perpendicular plate completes the posterior nasal wall. It fills the space between the pterygoid processes posteriorly and the ethmoid and maxillary bones anteriorly. One large and one or more smaller foramina are located in the bony palate just below the third molar teeth (Figure 2-10). The larger and more anterior foramen is the greater palatine foramen. The smaller lesser palatine foramina are located just posterior to the greater. These foramina transmit the greater (anterior) and lesser (posterior) palatine nerves and vessels respectively. The small orbital process of the perpendicular plate contributes to the floor of the orbit.

The Nasal Bones.   The paired nasal bones form the bony bridge of the nose (Figure 2-4). They articulate with each other at the midline as well as with the frontal bone, the perpendicular plate of the ethmoid, and the maxillary bones.

The Inferior Nasal Concha.   Unlike the superior and middle nasal conchae, the inferior nasal concha develops as a separate bone (Figure 2–13). It articulates with a ridge on the maxillary and palatine bones of the lateral nasal wall.

The Lacrimal Bone.   The lacrimal bone is a small, delicate, paired bone that forms part of the medial orbital wall (Figure 2–7). It lies anterior to the orbital plate of the ethmoid bone and forms the posterior margin of the fossa for the lacrimal sac and the nasolacrimal duct.

The Maxillary Bone.   The maxillary (maxillae) bones form the center of the face (Figure 2–4). They are fused medially and form portions of the palate, orbit, and nose. Each maxilla consists of a body and four processes, the zygomatic, frontal, palatine, and alveolar.

The body has four surfaces, the anterior (or malar), the posterior (or infratemporal), the orbital, and the nasal. The anterior surface extends from the midline of the face laterally to the zygomatic process. A foramen, the infraorbital foramen, is located in this surface just below the rim of the orbit. Two shallow depressions or fossae are located on the anterior surface. The incisive fossa is located above the roots of the incisive teeth. An elevation of the bone over the canine tooth lateral to the incisive fossa is called the canine eminence. The canine fossa is just lateral to the eminence. The anterior surface is bounded laterally by a ridge of bone that begins on the inferior border of the zygomatic process. The ridge curves downward from the base of the process ending at the alveolar process of the first molar tooth. It is called the jugal ridge. The posterior surface of the maxilla is that surface behind the jugal ridge. Several small alveolar canals perforate the posterior surface. They transmit the posterior superior alveolar vessels and nerves.

The orbital surface forms the floor of the orbit. It is marked by the infraorbital groove, which is continuous with the infraorbital foramen. The nasal surface forms the rest of the lateral wall of each nasal cavity. It has a ridge for articulation with the inferior nasal concha. The body of the maxilla contains the large maxillary sinus, which will be described with the paranasal sinuses.

The zygomatic process of the maxilla is a short, thick projection that articulates with the zygoma. The frontal process articulates with the nasal bone and completes the bridge of the nose. The alveolar processes hold the maxillary teeth. The anterior three fourths of the hard palate and the floor of the nasal cavities are formed from the palatine processes of the maxillary bones. Their median juncture is called the palatine raphe. The incisive foramen is located at the anterior end of the raphe behind the central incisors.

The Zygomatic Bones.   The zygomatic bones (singular zygoma) form the prominence of the cheeks (Figures 2–4 and 2–7). They also form the lateral wall and a portion of the floor of the orbit. Each bone has three processes—the frontal, maxillary, and temporal—which articulate with the zygomatic processes of the respective bones. The body of each bone is pierced by one or more small foramina, the zygomaticofacial foramina.

The Mandible.   The mandible consists of a horseshoe-shaped horizontal body and two vertical rami (Figure 2–15). The alveolar process on the upper margin of the body holds the mandibular teeth. The lower margin is smoothly rounded. The prominence of the chin is

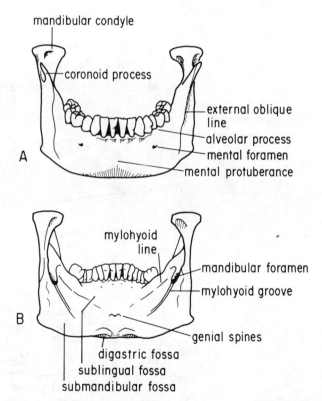

FIGURE 2–15   (A) anterior aspect of the mandible; (B) posterior aspect of the mandible.

the result of a slight bulge, the mental protuberance, located at the midline of the base of the body of the mandible. The mental foramen is located below the second bicuspid. It faces backward and slightly upward. A faint line begins at the mental foramen and passes posteriorly, becoming distinct in the area of the molar teeth and blending with the anterior edge of the ramus. This is the external oblique line.

The inner surface of the body of the mandible is marked by a line and several fossae (Figure 2-16). The mylohyoid line varies in prominence. It begins just below the third molars and curves downward, ending at the lower border of the center of the body. A depression below the line in the molar region is the submandibular fossa of the submandibular gland. Another depression above the line in the bicuspid region is the sublingual fossa of the sublingual gland. In the same area as the sublingual fossa but below the mylohyoid line on the inferior border of the mandible is a small depression, the digastric fossa.

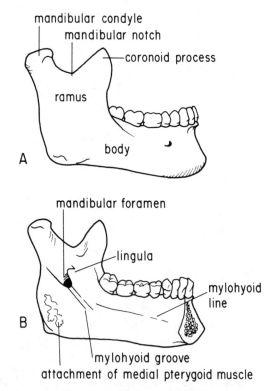

FIGURE 2-16   Lateral aspect of the mandible: (A) outer surface, (B) inner surface.

Four small spines are located anteriorly on either side of the midline of the body near the base. They are the mental (genial) spines, two superior and two inferior.

The vertical ramus is a flat, rectangular piece of bone that is continuous with the body of the mandible behind the molar teeth. The posterior inferior corner is the mandibular angle. The upper border presents a deep notch called the mandibular notch. The thin, flat, coronoid process projects anterior to the notch. The condylar process is posterior. The condylar process has a thin neck and a broad curved head, the mandibular condyle, for articulation with the glenoid fossa of the temporal bone.

The outer surface of the ramus of the mandible is slightly ridged for muscle attachment. The inner surface presents a foramen, the mandibular foramen, a little above the center. The mandibular foramen is the entrance to the mandibular canal, which opens onto the external surface of the mandible at the mental foramen. The mandibular foramen and canal transmit the mandibular nerve and vessels. The anterior lip of the foramen is marked by a sharp projection of bone, the lingula. A small groove, the mylohyoid groove, begins at the foramen and sweeps anteriorly toward the mylohyoid line. The inner surface of the angle of the mandible is very rough to allow muscular attachment.

The Hyoid Bone.   The hyoid bone is a small bone suspended between the styloid process and the thyroid cartilage of the larynx by ligaments (Figure 2–17). It is the point of origin or insertion for many of the muscles of the neck, tongue, and pharynx. It consists of a central body, two greater horns, and two lesser horns. The greater horns project posteriorly from the body. The lesser horns are small processes, projecting upward at the junction of the greater horns and the body and are attached by their tips to the styloid process by the stylohyoid ligament.

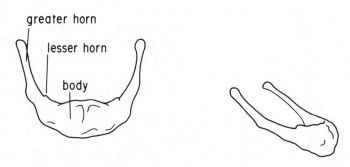

FIGURE 2–17   The hyoid bone.

Fossae and Landmarks

A number of fossae are delimited by the bones of the skull. The word *fossa* in this context means an area, not necessarily a depression.

The Cranial Fossae. The anterior, middle, and posterior cranial fossae are areas in the base of the cranial cavity. The anterior fossa is the area in front of the lesser wings of the sphenoid bone. The middle fossa is the area between the anterior surface of the petrous portion of the temporal bone and the lesser wings of the sphenoid bone. The posterior cranial fossa is the area of the cranial cavity behind the petrous portion of the temporal bone.

Temporal and Infratemporal Fossae (Figure 2-12). The temporal fossa is the area of origin of the temporalis muscle. The superior and posterior boundary is the superior temporal line. Anteriorly, it is limited by the back of the zygomatic process of the frontal bone. A horizontal plane passed between the upper border of the zygomatic arch and the skull would mark the approximate inferior limit. The area below this plane and behind the maxilla is the infratemporal fossa. The temporal and infratemporal fossae are continuous with one another.

Pterygopalatine Fossa.   (See Figure 2-12). If the mandible is removed and the skull is held at an angle so as to look behind the zygomatic arch, a triangular gap can be seen between the back of the maxilla and the superior end of the lateral pterygoid plate. This gap is called the pterygomaxillary fissure. The fissure leads into a small conical fossa, the pterygopalatine fossa. The fossa is triangular with the apex pointing down. The roof (base of the triangle) communicates with the inferior orbital fissure and so the orbit. The floor of the fossa (apex of the triangle) opens into the greater palatine canal. The lateral boundary of the fossa opens into the infratemporal fossa. The posterior and medial boundaries are bony. Each of these walls is pierced by two foramina. The posterior wall contains the foramen rotundum and the small pterygoid canal. The medial wall is perforated by the palato-vaginal canal, which leads to the pharynx and the sphenopalatine foramen, which communicates with the nasal cavity.

CHAPTER SUMMARY

Joints

I. Immovable
  A. Fibrous
    1. Sutures
      a. Held together by connective tissue
      b. Type of joint found between most of the bones of the skull
    2. *Schindylesis*
      a. *Tongue-in-groove-type joint secured with connective tissue*
      b. *Type of joint between ethmoid and vomer*
    3. *Gomphosis*
      a. *Peg-in-hole-type joint secured with connective tissue*
      b. *Type of joint between teeth and their bony sockets*
  B. Cartilaginous
    1. Held together by cartilage
    2. Type of joint found between bodies of vertebrae (intervertebral discs)
II. Movable
  A. Held together by muscles and ligaments
  B. Degree of movement depends on attachments of muscles and ligaments
  C. Ends of bones are covered with hyaline cartilage
  D. Articular disc is sometimes present
  E. Joint capsule surrounds the joint
  F. Joint is lubricated with a fluid called synovial fluid
  G. Examples of this kind of joint are the temporomandibular joint, craniovertebral joints, and vertebral articulations (except the intervertebral discs)

Bones

Bone	Parts or Surfaces	Grooves, Ridges and Processes	Foramina	Articulations
Cervical vertebrae	—	1. Transverse proc. 2. Spinous proc.	1. Vertebral foramen 2. Foramen transversarium	Vertebrae above and below
Atlas	—	Transverse proc.	1. Vertebral foramen 2. Foramen transversarium	Occipital condyles above, axis below
Axis	—	1. Transverse proc. 2. Spinous proc. 3. Odontoid proc.	1. Vertebral foramen 2. Foramen transversarium	Atlas above, 3rd. cervical vertebrae below
Frontal bone	1. *Squama* 2. *Intracranial* 3. *Intraorbital*	1. Zygomatic proc. 2. *Frontal crest* 3. *Nasal spine*	Supraorbital for.	Parietal bones, sphenoid, zygomatic, ethmoid, maxilla

Bones (continued)

Bone	Parts or Surfaces	Grooves, Ridges and Processes	Foramina	Articulations
Parietal	1. Extra-cranial 2. Intra-cranial	1. Temporal lines 2. Groove for middle meningeal a. 3. Groove for superior sagittal sinus	Parietal foramen	Contralateral parietal, frontal, temporal, occipital, sphenoid
Occipital	1. Squamous	1. Ext. occipital protuberance 2. Nuchal lines 3. Int. occipital protuberance 4. Groove for transverse sinus		
	2. Lateral			*Sphenoid, temporal, parietal*
	3. Condylar	5. Occipital condyles	1. Condylar foramen 2. Foramen magnum 3. Hypoglossal canal	
	4. Basilar	6. Pharyngeal tubercle		
Sphenoid	1. Greater wings		1. Foramen rotundum 2. Foramen ovale 3. Foramen spinosum 4. Optic canal	*Ethmoid, vomer, frontal temporal, parietal, occipital*

	2. Lesser wings
	3. Body
		1. Ant. clinoid proc.
		2. Middle and posterior clinoid processes
		3. Sella turcica
		4. Pterygoid processes
		  a. pterygoid hamulus
		  b. pterygoid fossa
		  c. scaphoid fossa		

Temporal	1. Squama	1. Groove for middle meningeal a. 2. Zygomatic process 3. Glenoid fossa 4. Articular tubercle	1. External auditory meatus	*Sphenoid, parietal, occipital*

Bones (continued)

Bone	Parts or Surfaces	Grooves, Ridges and Processes	Foramina	Articulations
	2. Mastoid	5. Mastoid process 6. Mastoid notch	2. Mastoid foramen	
	3. Styloid	7. Styloid process	3. Stylomastoid foramen	
	4. Petrous	8. Arcuate eminence	4. Internal auditory meatus	
		9. Depression for the trigeminal ganglion	5. Jugular foramen	
		10. Groove for the sigmoid sinus	6. Carotid canal	
Ethmoid	1. Cribriform plate 2. Perpendicular plate	1. Crista galli	Foramina for olfactory nerves	*Frontal, sphenoid, vomer, palatine*
	3. Labyrinths	2. Superior and middle nasal conchae		
Palatine	1. Horzontal plate			*Maxilla, ethmoid, sphenoid*
	2. Perpendicular plate	*Orbital process*	Greater and lesser palatine foramina	
Vomer				*Ethmoid, maxilla, sphenoid*
Nasal				*Frontal, maxilla, ethmoid*
Inferior nasal conchae				*Maxilla, palatine*
Lacrimal		1. Fossa for lacrimal sac 2. Nasolacrimal duct		*Ethmoid, frontal, maxilla*
Maxilla	A. Body 1. Anterior sur. (Malar)	1. Incisive fossa 2. Canine eminence 3. Canine fossa 4. Jugal ridge	1. Infraorbital foramen	

Bones (continued)

Bone	Parts or Surfaces	Grooves, Ridges and Processes	Foramina	Articulations
	2. Posterior sur. (Infratemporal)		2. Foramina for the posterior superior alveolar vessels and nerves	
	3. Orbital sur.	5. Infraorbital grv.		*Frontal, nasal, lacrimal, ethmoid, zygomatic, palatine, sphenoid, inferior nasal concha*
	4. nasal sur.	6. Ridge for inferior nasal conchae		
	B. Palatal sur.	7. Palatine process	3. Incisive for.	
	C. Other processes of the body	8. Zygomatic process		
		9. Frontal process		
		10. Alveolar processes		
Zygomatic	Body	1. Frontal proc.	Zygomaticofacial for.	*Frontal, maxilla, temporal*
		2. Maxillary proc.		
		3. Temporal proc.		
Mandible	A. Body			
	1. Outer sur.	1. Mental protuberance	1. Mental foramen	*Temporal*
		2. External oblique line		
	2. Inner sur.	3. Mylohyoid line		
		4. Submandibular fossa		
		5. Sublingual fossa		
		6. Digastric fossa		
		7. Mental (genial) spines		
	3. Superior sur.	8. Alveolar processes		
	B. Ramus	9. Coronoid proc.		
		10. Condylar proc.		
		11. Mandibular notch		

Bones (continued)

Bone	Parts or Surfaces	Grooves, Ridges and Processes	Foramina	Articulations
	Inner sur.	12. Lingula 13. Mylohyoid groove	2. Mandibular foramen	
Hyoid	1. Body 2. Greater horns 3. Lesser horns			Suspended between styloid proc. and thyroid cartilage by ligaments

Sutures of the Skull

Suture	Bones Involved
Coronal	Frontal, both parietal bones
Sagittal	Parietal bones
Lambdoid	Parietal bones and occipital bone

STUDY EXERCISES

1. What are the two types of immovable joints?

2. Name three types of fibrous joints found in the head.

3. The intervertebral discs are examples of what type of immovable joint?

4. *Besides the ability to move, what are the differences between movable and immovable joints?*

5. Name the bone with which each of the following structures is associated: Pterygoid process, digastric fossa, infraorbital foramen, external occipital protuberance, crista galli, coronoid process, styloid process, foramen rotundum, mylohyoid line, superior and middle nasal conchae, zygomaticofacial foramena, incisive fossa, lesser palatine foramena, mastoid process, lingula, foramen ovale, odontoid process, stylomastoid foramen, hypoglossal canal.

6. *Name the bones that make up the bony nasal septum.*

7. With what three bones does the zygoma articulate?

8. *Name the three sutures of the calvaria, and state which bones unite to form the sutures.*

9. *Describe the locations of the anterior, middle, and posterior cranial fossae.*

10. Describe the limits of the temporal and infratemporal fossae.

11. *Diagram the pterygomandibular fossa showing the walls and foramina. Refer to the description in the text.*

3

THE
MUSCULAR
SYSTEM

LEARNING OBJECTIVES

At the conclusion of this chapter, the student should be able to:

1. Give the names, innervation, and group actions of the supra- and infrahyoid muscles.
2. Give the names, innervation, and actions of the muscles of facial expression.
3. Give the names, innervation, origin, insertion, and actions of the muscles of mastication.
4. Describe the *origin, insertion,* innervation, and actions of the pharyngeal muscles.
5. Give the *origin, insertion,* action, and innervation of the extrinsic muscles of the tongue.
6. *Describe the process of deglutition.*

The muscles of the head and neck may be divided into regional and functional groups. While each muscle is described individually, virtually no muscle acts alone. Rather, muscles act in groups as synergists and/or antagonists to one another, maintaining posture and carrying out the minute-by-minute commands of the central nervous system.

MUSCLES OF THE NECK

The Posterior and Suboccipital Neck Muscles

Except for the trapezius, the muscles of the posterior neck, suboccipital, and anterior vertebral regions are not described individually. The reader is referred to one of the fine general anatomy texts listed in the references for more information.

The posterior neck and suboccipital muscles rotate and extend the head and bend the cervical spine posteriorly and laterally.

Trapezius. The trapezius is the most superficial muscle of the posterior neck (Figure 3–1). It functions mainly as a fixator of the arm, but it is briefly described here because it forms a smooth transition of the neck to the shoulder and back and moves the head if the attachment in the shoulder is fixed. The trapezius originates from the medial one third of the superior nuchal line, the external occipital protuberance, and the ligamentum nuchae. The latter is a very tough ligament at the midline of the neck that joins the spinous processes of the cervical vertebrae and serves as attachment for some neck muscles. The trapezius inserts into the posterior border of the lateral one third of the clavicle and the shoulder. With the shoulder fixed, the muscle draws the head backward and laterally. Innervation is from the spinal accessory or eleventh cranial nerve.

Anterior Vertebral Muscles

The anterior vertebral muscles are located on the anterior surface of the cervical vertebral column. These muscles lie between the skull and atlas and between the individual vertebrae. They bend the head and neck forward and laterally. They are innervated by cervical segmental nerves, that is, by branches of the spinal nerves that emerge from the spinal cord between the cervical vertebrae.

Lateral Neck Muscles

The lateral neck muscles are located on each side of the vertebral column.

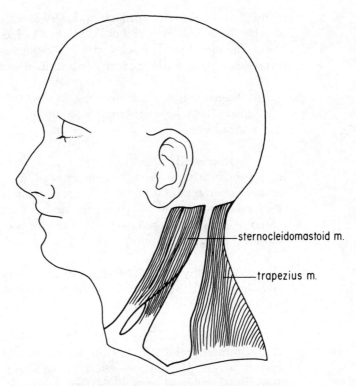

FIGURE 3-1   Lateral neck muscles.

Sternocleidomastoid.   The most prominent and superficial lateral neck muscle is the sternocleidomastoid (Figure 3-1). It arises by two heads from the top of the sternum and medial one third of the clavicle. The two heads converge and insert on the mastoid process and lateral portion of the superior nuchal line. The muscle pulls the mastoid process down and rotates the chin upward to the opposite side. It is innervated by the spinal accessory or eleventh cranial nerve.

The Scalene and Levator Scapulae Muscles.   The anterior, middle, and posterior scalene muscles and the levator scapulae muscle are also lateral neck muscles. However, their primary actions are on the first and second ribs and shoulder girdle. In addition, they may flex the neck and bend it laterally.

Infrahyoid Muscles

The four paired infrahyoid muscles are located below the hyoid bone in the front of the neck (Figure 3-2). They are thin, strap-like muscles that lie on the sides and front of the trachea. Their names give their origin and insertion. Their collective action is to pull down or depress the hyoid bone or thyroid cartilage during swallowing and speech. They also fix the hyoid bone or hold it firmly in place so that the muscles above, the suprahyoid muscles, may act on the mandible. Innervation is through the cervical plexus, which is described with the nervous system.

Sternohyoid.   The sternohyoid muscle is the most superficial. It originates from the manubrium of the sternum and inserts on the body of the hyoid bone.

Omohyoid.   The omohyoid muscle has two bellies. The inferior belly arises from the scapula and ends in an intermediate tendon behind the origin of the sternocleidomastoid muscle. Here the superior belly takes origin and inserts on the body of the hyoid lateral to the sternohyoid muscle. The intermediate tendon is held to the clavicle by a tendinous sling, the length of which is quite variable.

Sternothyroid.   The sternothyroid muscle lies beneath the sternohyoid. It arises from the sternum and inserts on the side of the thyroid cartilage of the larynx.

Thyrohyoid.   The thyrohyoid is considered to be an extension of the sternothyroid. It runs from the insertion of that muscle to the inferior border of the greater horn of the hyoid. If the hyoid bone is fixed, the thyrohyoid can pull the larynx upward. If the larynx is fixed, the muscle pulls down on the hyoid bone.

Suprahyoid Muscles

The suprahyoid muscles are located between the hyoid bone and the mandible (Figure 3-2). They act, therefore, on one or both of those bones during speech, chewing, and swallowing. They also fix the hyoid bone superiorly while the infrahyoid muscles function.

Digastric.   If the chin is raised and the muscles under it viewed, the digastric muscle is the most superficial. Each digastric has two bellies. The anterior belly arises from the digastric fossa of the mandible and ends in an intermediate tendon, which is attached by a tendinous sling to the greater horn of the hyoid bone near its junction with the body. The posterior belly arises from the intermediate tendon and inserts on the mastoid notch or groove. The anterior belly draws the hyoid bone forward and is innervated by the mylohyoid branch of the fifth cranial nerve, the trigeminal. The posterior belly pulls the hyoid bone backward and is innervated by a branch of the seventh cranial nerve, the facial.

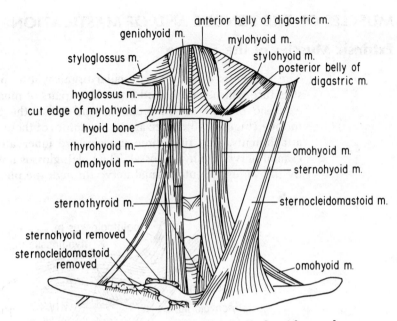

FIGURE 3–2 Suprahyoid and infrahyoid muscles.

Mylohyoid. The mylohyoid muscle forms the floor of the mouth. It originates from the mylohyoid line on each side of the mandible. Most of the fibers meet in a medial raphe. The most posterior fibers insert on the upper margin of the body of the hyoid bone. This arrangement means that the posterolateral margins of the muscle are free. The mylohyoid elevates the floor of the mouth and the hyoid bone during swallowing. It is innervated by the mylohyoid branch of the trigeminal nerve.

Geniohyoid. The geniohyoid muscles are two small bands arising from the genial tubercles and inserting on the upper border of the body of the hyoid bone. They lie on top of the mylohyoid muscle on either side of the midline of the floor of the mouth. The geniohyoids may elevate the hyoid bone or depress the mandible, depending on which attachment is fixed. They are innervated by the first cervical nerve, which travels with the hypoglossal or twelfth cranial nerve.

Stylohyoid. The stylohyoid muscle lies superficial to the posterior belly of the digastric muscle. As its name implies, it originates from the styloid process of the temporal bone and inserts on the hyoid bone near the tendon of the digastric. Like the posterior digastric, the stylohyoid draws the hyoid bone backward and is innervated by a branch of the facial nerve.

MUSCLES OF THE TONGUE AND OF MASTICATION

Extrinsic Muscles of the Tongue

The tongue is a complex muscular organ whose internal or intrinsic structure will be considered later. Four pairs of muscles comprise the extrinsic or external musculature and make the tongue extremely mobile (Figure 3–3). Once again, the names of these muscles give their attachments. The first three muscles are innervated by the twelfth cranial nerve, the hypoglossal. The palatoglossus muscle is innervated by the vagus or tenth cranial nerve through the pharyngeal plexus.

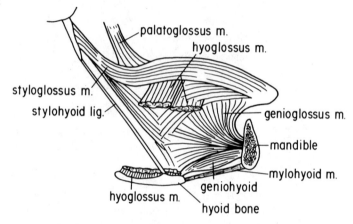

FIGURE 3–3   Extrinsic muscles of the tongue.

Genioglossus.   The genioglossus arises from the superior genial tubercles of the mandible and fans out vertically. Most of the fibers blend with the intrinsic muscles of the tongue from the tip of the root. The most posterior fibers insert on the body of the hyoid bone. The posterior fibers protrude the tongue, while the anterior fibers retract it.

Hyoglossus.   The hyoglossus arises from the greater horn and body of the hyoid and inserts by two heads on the side of the tongue. It depresses the sides of the tongue and retracts it.

Styloglossus.   The styloglossus muscle originates on the styloid process. Like the hyoglossus, it splits into two heads for insertion. One head inserts at the side of the tongue between the two heads of the hyoglossus muscle. The other head blends with the intrinsic muscle of the side of the tongue from the root to the tip. The styloglossus retracts and elevates the tongue.

Palatoglossus. The palatoglossus extends from the under-surface of the soft palate to the side of the root of the tongue. It elevates the back of the tongue.

Muscles of Mastication

Four muscles, the temporalis, masseter, medial, and lateral pterygoids, are largely responsible for the chewing action of the jaws and are called the muscles of mastication. They are innervated by the trigeminal nerve. The supra- and infrahyoid muscles aid the major muscles and are sometimes called accessory muscles of mastication.

Temporalis. The temporalis muscle is covered by a tough sheet of connective tissue called the *temporal fascia*. The muscle originates from the entire temporal fossa and the temporal fascia (Figure 3–4). The anterior and superior fibers are vertical, while the posterior fibers are almost horizontal. The temporalis converges into an insertion on the medial aspect of the coronoid process of the mandible as well as the anterior and posterior borders of the process. Some fibers also insert on the anterior border of the ramus of the mandible to a point just behind the last molar tooth. The anterior and superior fibers elevate the mandible. The posterior fibers pull the mandible posteriorly.

Masseter. The masseter has a superficial and a deep origin (Figure 3–4). Superficial fibers arise from the inferior border of the anterior two-thirds of the zygomatic arch. The deeper fibers arise from the inside of the posterior one-third of the zygomatic arch. The fibers converge and form a very powerful muscle that inserts on the angle and lower half of the lateral surface of the ramus and a portion of the upper half, including the lateral surface of the coronoid process. The masseter is a powerful elevator of the mandible.

Medial and Lateral Pterygoids. The medial and lateral ptery-goid muscles, acting together and in concert with the contralateral pterygoid muscles, are responsible for the rotation and grinding motion of the jaws (Figure 3–5).

The lateral pterygoid originates by two heads. The upper head arises from the infratemporal surface of the sphenoid bone. The lower head arises from the lateral surface of the lateral pterygoid plate. The fibers converge and end on the head of the mandible, articular disc, and temporomandibular joint capsule. The muscle assists in opening the mouth by pulling the head of the mandible forward. If the lateral pterygoid of one side contracts, it rotates the mandible on a vertical axis through the mandibular condyle of the opposite side.

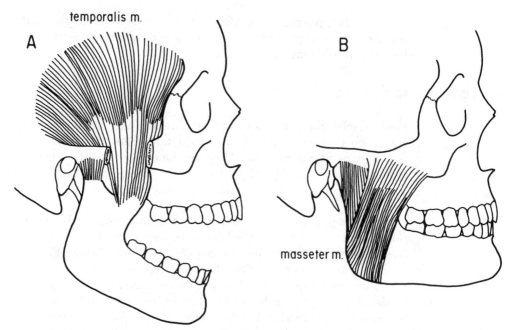

FIGURE 3–4   (A) attachments of the temporalis muscle; (B) attachments of the masseter muscle.

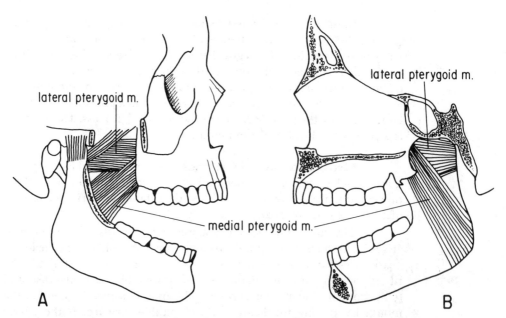

FIGURE 3–5   Medial and lateral pterygoid muscles: (A) lateral aspect, (B) medial aspect.

The medial pterygoid has a superficial and deep origin. Superficial fibers from the maxillary tuberosity meet deep fibers from the medial surface of the lateral pterygoid plate. The muscle inserts on the angle of the medial surface of the ramus of the mandible below the mandibular foramen and posterior to the mylohyoid groove. The medial pterygoid elevates and protrudes the mandible.

THE TEMPOROMANDIBULAR JOINT AND ITS MOVEMENTS

The temporomandibular joint (TMJ) is a synovial joint between the condyle of the mandible and the glenoid fossa of the temporal bone. The fossa and condyle are covered with fibrocartilage. An articular disc divides the joint cavity into upper and lower parts (Figure 3–6). The disc is attached anteriorly and posteriorly to the surrounding joint capsule and medially and laterally to the condyle. This ensures that the disc and condyle move together.

The capsule surrounds the joint cavity (Figure 3–7). It attaches to the rim of the glenoid fossa and the neck of the condyle. It is reinforced laterally by the temporomandibular or lateral ligament. Two other ligaments are associated with the joint. The sphenomandibular ligament is a thickening in the fascia that connects the spine of the sphenoid to the lingula of the mandible. The stylomandibular ligament extends between the styloid process and the posterior border of the ramus of the mandible near the angle. These last two ligaments are considered accessory ligaments, and their role is obscure.

Table 3–1 is a summary of the movements of the TMJ and the muscles that produce the movement. Figure 3–8 is a diagram of the directions of pull of these muscles. The jaw can be opened (depressed),

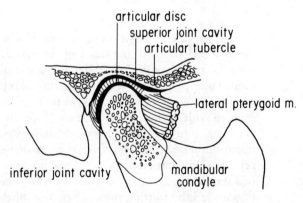

FIGURE 3–6   Sagittal section through the temporomandibular joint.

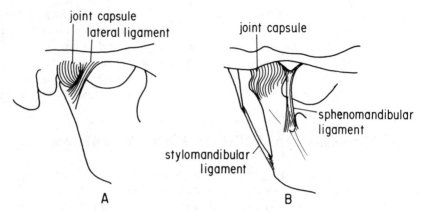

FIGURE 3–7   The temporomandibular joint: (A) lateral aspect, (B) medial aspect.

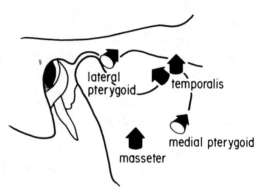

FIGURE 3–8   Diagram of the direction of pull of the muscles of mastication.

closed (elevated), protruded, retruded, and displaced laterally. When the jaw is depressed, the head of the mandible slides forward and up onto the articular tubercle. When the jaw is elevated, the opposite movement takes place, and the head of the mandible comes to rest against the posterior wall of the glenoid fossa (Figure 3–6). When the jaw is opened wide, a sharp blow or muscle spasm can cause it to ride over the articular tubercle and become dislocated. Dislocation is not an uncommon occurrence. Often, the person can reduce the joint himself, returning the mandible to its normal position. Sometimes the assistance of another person is required. The mandible must be pushed downward, by putting pressure on the third molars, and backward by elevating the chin. This allows the head of the condyle to slip back over the tubercle to its proper position.

TABLE 3–1. Muscles Producing Movement at the Temporomandibular Joint

Movement	Muscle
Depression of the Mandible	Lateral Pterygoids Assisted by Suprahyoids
Elevation of the Mandible	Temporalis, Masseter. Medial Pterygoid
Protrusion of the Mandible	Medial and Lateral Pterygoids
Retraction of the Mandible	Temporalis Assisted by the Masseter, Digastric, and Geniohyoid
Lateral Movements of the Mandible	Medial and Lateral Pterygoids of Each Side Acting Alternately

While certain movements are attributed to individual muscles or groups of muscles, it must be kept in mind that the complex movements of the TMJ are the result of all the muscles working in a coordinated, alternating pattern. Damage to the articular disc may cause clicking (crepitus) and pain in the joint.

MUSCLES OF FACIAL EXPRESSION

The muscles of facial expression are small, subcutaneous muscles that form the sphinctors of the eyes and mouth and, by wrinkling the skin, result in all our varied facial expressions (Figure 3–9). Many of these muscles have no bony attachments but arise and insert into skin or other muscles. They are all innervated by the seventh cranial nerve, the facial nerve.

Muscles of the Scalp

Frontalis.   The frontalis is a thin sheet of muscle that originates from the fascia of the scalp, the galea aponeurotica. It extends from the region of the anterior scalp to the skin above the supraorbital area. It pulls the scalp forward, wrinkles the skin of the forehead, and raises the eyebrows.

Occipitalis.   The occipitalis is the posterior homologue of the frontalis. It arises from the occipital bone and inserts into the galea aponeurotica. It pulls the scalp backward.

Muscles of the Ears

Anterior, Posterior, and Superior Auricular Muscles.   The anterior auricular muscle is quite small and originates from the temporal fascia. The fibers end on the helix of the ear and draw the ear forward. The posterior auricular muscle arises from the mastoid process and inserts on the posterior aspect of the ear. It draws the ear backward.

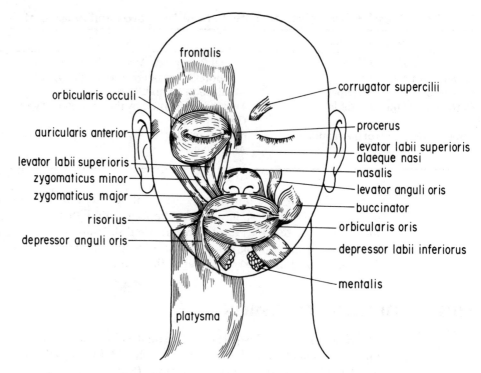

FIGURE 3-9   Muscles of facial expression.

The superior auricular muscle runs from the galea aponeurotica to the pinna of the ear and elevates the pinna. All of these muscles vary greatly in size and degree of control that can be exerted by the individual.

Muscles of the Eyes

Orbicularis Oculi.   The orbicularis oculi muscle encircles the eye. It arises and inserts medially from the lacrimal bone, frontal bone, and frontal process of the maxilla. It may be divided into orbital and palpebral (eyelid) parts. Together, they close the eye.

Procerus.   The procerus is a tiny muscle running from the bridge of the nose to the skin of the root of the nose. It draws the skin of the forehead down.

Corrugator Supercilii.   The corrugator is another tiny muscle. Arising at the medial end of the superciliary arch, it inserts into the skin above the orbital arch. Contraction causes the eyebrows to be drawn down and in.

Muscles of the Nose

Nasalis. The nasalis muscle is sometimes divided into two parts, the compressor naris and the depressor septi. The compressor arises from the incisive fossa and inserts into the fascia of the nose. It compresses the nostrils, making the opening wider. The depressor portion arises from the same area but inserts into the base of the nasal septum. It assists in widening the nasal aperture.

Muscles of the Mouth

Orbicularis Oris. The fibers of the orbicularis oris muscle form the lips and encircle the mouth. Some fibers originate from the alveolar processes of the maxilla and mandible and insert into the substance of the lip. However, many of the fibers of the orbicularis come from the other muscles that insert on the mouth. The muscle closes and protrudes the lips and shapes them during speech.

Levator Labii Superioris Alaeque Nasi. Levator labii superioris alaeque nasi is a much smaller muscle than its name would indicate. It arises from the frontal process of the maxilla. The tiny slip of muscle divides into a portion that inserts on the ala of the nose and a portion that ends on the upper lip. It elevates the lip and dilates the naris.

Levator Labii Superioris. Levator labii superioris is lateral to the alaeque nasi. Its fibers extend from the orbital rim above the infraorbital foramen to the upper lip. It elevates the lip.

Levator Anguli Oris. Levator anguli oris lies beneath both the alaeque nasi and levator labii superioris. It arises from the canine fossa just below the infraorbital foramen and inserts into the angle of the mouth, which it elevates.

Zygomaticus Major and Minor. The zygomaticus major and minor both arise from the zygoma, the minor at the maxillary suture and the major more laterally. The minor inserts on the upper lip lateral to the alaeque nasi insertion. The major ends at the corner of the mouth. Zygomaticus minor elevates the upper lip, while zygomaticus major elevates the corner of the mouth.

Buccinator. The buccinator forms the substance of the cheek. It arises from the alveolar processes of the maxilla and mandible and the pterygomandibular raphe. The pterygomandibular raphe is a group of connective tissue fibers stretching from the pterygoid hamulus to the posterior end of the mylohyoid line of the mandible. The buccinator inserts into and blends with the orbicularis oris at the corner of the mouth. These fibers are a major portion of the substance of the lips. The buccinator compresses the cheek against the teeth, keeping food between the teeth during chewing. It also retracts and raises the angle of the mouth.

Risorius.   The risorius is a very small muscle arising from the fascia over the buccinator and inserting at the corner of the mouth. It compresses the cheek and pulls the angle of the mouth laterally.

Depressor Anguli Oris.   The depressor anguli oris arises from the anterior end of the external oblique line of the mandible and ends at the angle of the mouth. It depresses the angle of the mouth.

Depressor Labii Inferioris.   Depressor labii inferioris originates from the external oblique line of the mandible deep to the depressor anguli oris. It inserts into the orbicularis oris and the lower lip, which it depresses.

Mentalis.   The mentalis arises from a slight depression below the mandibular incisor teeth and ends in the skin of the chin. It protrudes the lower lip.

Platysma.   The platysma is a very thin sheet of muscle that begins in the fascia of the shoulder and upper chest. The fibers pass upward and end on the lower border of the mandible and muscles and skin of the mouth and lower face. It draws the outer part of the mouth and skin of the chin downward as in a pout.

MUSCLES OF THE SOFT PALATE AND THE PHARYNX

Muscles of the Soft Palate

There are three muscles that make up the substance of the soft palate. Their collective function is to elevate the soft palate during swallowing, closing off the nasopharynx above from the oropharynx below.

Levator Veli Palatini.   The levator veli palatini arises from the undersurface of the petrous part of the temporal bone and the auditory (Eustachian) tube. It ends in the aponeurosis of the soft palate (Figure 3–10). It elevates the soft palate during swallowing. Innervation is via the pharyngeal plexus.

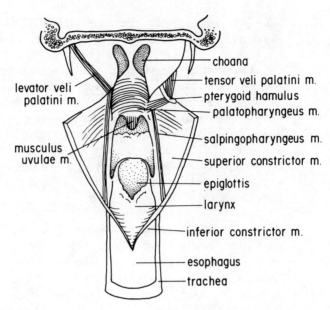

choana
tensor veli palatini m.
pterygoid hamulus
palatopharyngeus m.
levator veli palatini m.
salpingopharyngeus m.
superior constrictor m.
musculus uvulae m.
epiglottis
larynx
inferior constrictor m.
esophagus
trachea

FIGURE 3–10 Posterior view of the open pharynx showing larynx and nasal cavities.

Tensor Veli Palatini.   The tensor veli palatini arises from the scaphoid fossa, sphenoid spine, and Eustachian tube (Figure 3-10). The tendon passes upward and hooks around the hamulus of the pterygoid to insert horizontally into the soft palate. When it contracts, the muscle pulls laterally on each side of the soft palate, tensing it. The tensor receives its nervous supply from the trigeminal nerve.

Musculus Uvuli.   The musculus uvuli arise from the posterior nasal spine (Figure 3-10). They have no insertion but form the uvula. Upon contraction, the uvula shortens. The uvula is innervated by the pharyngeal plexus.

Muscles of the Pharynx

The pharynx is a muscular tube that begins at the base of the skull and ends in the esophagus and larynx. It consists of three overlapping constrictor muscles and three smaller muscles, all of which function in swallowing or deglutition. The pharynx may be divided into three functional areas. The nasopharynx is that area of the pharynx posterior to the nasal cavities above the plane of the soft palate. The oropharynx is that area below the nasopharynx and behind the oral cavity. It extends inferiorly to the level of the hyoid bone. The laryngopharynx is that portion of the pharynx below the hyoid bone which contains the larynx.

Superior Constrictor.   The superior constrictor muscle is a thin sheet that arises from the pterygoid hamulus, posterior margin of the medial pterygoid plate, pterygomandibular raphe, and posterior end of the mylohyoid line on the inner surface of the mandible (Figures 3–11 and 3–12). The fibers from each side pass posteriorly and upwards and unite in a median raphe. The superior end of the raphe attaches to the pharyngeal tubercle of the occipital bone. The space between the superior edge of the muscle and base of the skull is closed by the pharyngobasilar fascia.

Middle Constrictor.   Fibers of the middle constrictor muscle arise from the greater and lesser horns of the hyoid bone and the lower edge of the stylohyoid ligament. The stylohyoid ligament extends from the tip of the styloid process to the hyoid bone. Like the superior constrictor, the fibers from each side pass backward and unite at the median raphe (Figure 3–11 and 3–12). The upper fibers of the middle constrictor curve upward and overlap the lower fibers of the superior constrictor. The lower fibers of the middle constrictor curve downward and will be overlapped by the inferior constrictor muscle.

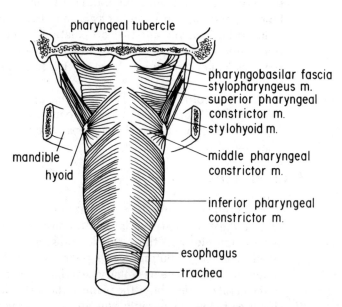

FIGURE 3–11   Posterior view of the pharyngeal constrictor muscles.

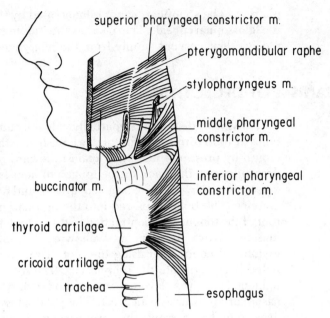

FIGURE 3-12   Lateral view of the pharyngeal constrictor muscles.

Inferior Constrictor.   The inferior constrictor is the thickest of the three pharyngeal muscles (Figures 3-11 and 3-12). It arises from the lateral portion of the larynx, the cricoid and thyroid cartilages. As with the other constrictors, the fibers of both sides meet at the posterior midline in the median raphe. The inferior fibers blend with the muscle coats of the esophagus. The superior fibers curve upward to overlap the middle constrictor.

All three constrictors are innervated by the pharyngeal plexus. They narrow the pharynx during swallowing.

Palatopharyngeus.   The palatopharyngeus muscle arises from the soft palate and inserts on the thyroid cartilage and pharyngeal aponeurosis. It narrows the oropharyngeal opening and closes off the nasopharynx (Figure 3-10).

Salpingopharyngeus.   The salpingopharyngeus muscle takes origin from the cartilage of the Eustachian tube and blends with the palatopharyngeus (Figure 3-10). It helps elevate the nasopharynx.

Stylopharyngeus.   The stylopharyngeus muscle arises from the base of the styloid process and inserts on the thyroid cartilage and side of the pharynx (Figures 3-11 and 3-12). It elevates and dilates the pharynx. The stylopharyngeus is innervated by the ninth cranial nerve, the glossopharyngeal. The palato- and salpingopharyngeus muscles receive their nervous supply from the pharyngeal plexus.

MECHANISM OF DEGLUTITION

Swallowing or deglutition is partially voluntary and partially reflex. The bolus of food formed on the tongue is pushed to the posterior part of the mouth by pressing the tongue against the hard palate. The soft palate descends onto the back of the tongue to help form the bolus. Simultaneously, the hyoid bone is pulled upward and fixed by the suprahyoid muscles. The bolus is passed into the oropharynx by elevation of the root of the tongue and contraction of the styloglossus and palatoglossus muscles. Now the act of swallowing becomes involuntary. The mylohyoid contracts, raising the root of the tongue and causing it to bulge backward into the oropharynx. The soft palate is elevated and tightened by the levator and tensor veli palatini muscles. The nasopharynx is now sealed off. The palatoglossus and palatopharyngeus muscles narrow the oropharyngeal opening. The superior constrictor muscle contracts, forcing the bolus downward. At the same time, the larynx and pharynx are pulled upwards by the stylo-, salpingo-, and palatopharyngeus muscles and the thyrohyoid muscles. Muscles in the larynx close its entrance and, with the epiglottis, form a smooth surface over which the bolus can slide without entering the airway. Contractions of the middle and, finally, the inferior constrictor muscles force the food into the esophagus.

CHAPTER SUMMARY

Muscles

Muscle	Origin	Insertion	Nerve	Action
Trapezius	Medial 1/3 sup. nuchal line, Ext. occipital protub., lig. nuchae	Lateral 1/3 of clavicle and shoulder	Spinal access. (XI)	With shoulder fixed, it draws the head back and laterally
Sternocleido-mastoid	Sternum and clavicle	Mastoid process and lat. superior nuchal line	Spinal access. (XI)	Pulls head back and rotates chin up to opposite side
Infrahyoid			Cervical plexus	Depress the hyoid bone or thyroid cartilage during swallowing and speech. Fix the hyoid bone.
1. Sternohyoid	Sternum	Body of hyoid		
2. Omohyoid				
inferior	Scapula	Intermediate tendon		
superior	Intermediate tendon	Body of hyoid		
3. Sternothyroid	Sternum	Thyroid cartilage		
4. Thyrohyoid	Insertion of sternothyroid	Bottom of the greater horn of hyoid		
Suprahyoid				
1. Digastric				
anterior	Digastric fossa	Intermediate tendon	Mylohyoid br. of trigeminal (V)	Draws the hyoid forward
posterior	Intermediate tendon	Mastoid notch	Facial (VII)	Draws the hyoid backward
2. Mylohyoid	Mylohyoid line	Median raphe, body of hyoid	Mylohyoid br. of trigeminal (V)	Elevates the floor of the mouth during swallowing
3. Geniohyoid	Genial spines	Body of hyoid	Cervical plexus	Elevates hyoid or depresses mandible
4. Stylohyoid	Styloid process	Hyoid near digastric tendon	Facial (VII)	Draws the hyoid backward
Extrinsic tongue				
1. Genioglossus	Genial spines	Intrinsic muscles of tongue and hyoid bone	Hypoglossal (XII)	Posterior fibers protrude tongue, anterior fibers retract it
2. Hyoglossus	Greater horn and body of hyoid bone	By two heads on side of tongue	Hypoglossal (XII)	Depresses sides of tongue and retracts it

Muscles (continued)

Muscle	Origin	Insertion	Nerve	Action
3. Styloglossus	*Styloid process*	*Two heads: Side of tongue betw. hyoglossus, side of tongue from root to tip*	Hypoglossal (XII)	Retracts and elevates tongue
4. Palatoglossus	*Undersurface of soft palate*	*Side of root of tongue*	Vagus (X)	Elevates back of tongue
Muscles of mastication				
1. Temporalis	Temporal fossa and fascia	Coronoid process and anterior border of the ramus of the mandible	Trigeminal (V)	Elevates and re-tracts mandible
2. Masseter superficial	Bottom of ant. 2/3 zygomatic arch	Lateral surface of ramus of man-dible including coronoid pro-cess and angle blends with superficial	Trigeminal (V)	Elevates mandible
deep	Inside of post. 1/3 of zygomatic arch			
3. Lateral pterygoid upper head	Infratemporal surface of sphenoid bone	Neck of the condylar pro-cess, articular disc, TMJ joint capsule	Trigeminal (V)	Opens the mouth by pull-ing the head of the mandible forward, rotates the mandible
lower head	Lateral surface of lateral pterygoid plate	Merges with upper head		
4. Medial pterygoid superficial	Maxillary tuberosity	Angle of mandi-ble on medial surface of ramus below the man-dibular for. and behind the mylohyoid line	Trigeminal (V)	Elevates and protrudes the mandible

Muscles (continued)

Muscle	Origin	Insertion	Nerve	Action
deep	Medial surface of lateral pterygoid plate	Blends with superficial part		
Muscles of facial expression				
1. Frontalis	Fascia of scalp	Skin of supra-orbital region	Facial (VII)	Wrinkles skin of forehead, raises eyebrows
2. Occipitalis	Occipital bone	Galea aponeurotica	Facial (VII)	Pulls scalp backward
3. Auricular				
anterior	Temporal fascia	Helix of the ear	Facial (VII)	Draws ear forward
posterior	Mastoid process	Back of the ear	Facial (VII)	Draws the ear backward
superior	Galea aponeurotica	Pinna of ear	Facial (VII)	Elevates the pinna
3. Orbicularis oculi	Lacrimal bone, frontal bone, Frontal proc. of max.	Encircles the eye and inserts on the bones of origin	Facial (VII)	Closes the eye
4. Procerus	Bridge of nose	Skin of root of nose	Facial (VII)	Draws the skin of the forehead down
5. Corrugator supercilii	Superciliary arch near nose	Skin above the arch	Facial (VII)	Draws the eyebrows together
6. Nasalis				
compressor	Incisive fossa	Fascia of nose	Facial (VII)	Compresses nostrils, making opening wider
depressor septi		Base of nasal septum		Assists the compressor
7. Orbicularis oris	Alveolar proc. of maxilla and mandible	Substance of the lip	Facial (VII)	Closes and protrudes the lips, shapes lips during speech
8. Levator labii superioris alaeque nasi	Frontal proc. of max.	Ala. of nose, upper lip	Facial (VII)	Elevates lip, dilates naris
9. Levator labii superioris	Orbital rim above infra-orbital for.	Upper lip	Facial (VII)	Elevates lip

Muscles (continued)

Muscle	Origin	Insertion	Nerve	Action
10. Levator anguli oris	Canine fossa	Angle of mouth	Facial (VII)	Elevates the angle of the mouth
11. Zygomaticus major	Zygoma at suture with maxilla	Corner of mouth	Facial (VII)	Elevates corner of mouth
12. Zygomaticus minor	Zygoma lateral to major	Upper lip	Facial (VII)	Elevates upper lip
13. Buccinator	Pterygomandibular raphe, alveolar procs. of mand. and max.	Orbicularis oris at corner of mouth	Facial (VII)	Forms substance of cheek, compresses cheek against teeth, retracts and raises angle of mouth
14. Risorius	Fascia over buccinator	Corner of mouth	Facial (VII)	Compresses cheek, pulls angle of mouth laterally
15. Depressor anguli oris	Ant. end of ext. oblique line	Angle of mouth	Facial (VII)	Depresses angle of mouth
16. Depressor labii inferioris	Ext. oblique line deep to depressor anguli oris	Orbicularis oris and lower lip	Facial (VII)	Depresses lower lip
17. Mentalis	Body of mandible below incisors	Skin of chin	Facial (VII)	Protrudes lower lip
18. Platysma	Fascia of shoulder and upper chest	Lower border of mandible, muscles and skin of lower face	Facial (VII)	Draws down the outer part of the mouth and skin of the chin as in a pout

Muscles of the soft palate

Muscle	Origin	Insertion	Nerve	Action
1. Levator veli palatini	Undersurface of petrous temporal bone and auditory tube	Aponeurosis of soft palate	Pharyngeal plexus	Elevates soft palate during swallowing
2. Tensor veli palatini	Scaphoid fossa, spine of sphenoid, auditory tube	Soft palate	Trigeminal (V)	Tenses soft palate
3. Musculus uvuli	Posterior nasal spine	None, forms uvula	Pharyngeal plexus	Shortens uvula

Muscles (continued)

Muscle	Origin	Insertion	Nerve	Action
Muscles of the pharynx				
1. Superior constrictor	Pterygoid hamulus, posterior margin of medial pterygoid plate, pterygomandibular raphe, posterior end of mylohyoid line	Median raphe, pharyngeal tubercle	Pharyngeal plexus	Narrow pharynx during swallowing
2. Middle constrictor	Greater and lesser horns of hyoid, lower edge of stylohyoid lig.	Median raphe	Pharyngeal plexus	Narrows pharynx during swallowing
3. Inferior constrictor	Lateral portion of larynx, thyroid, and cricoid cartilages	Median raphe, blends with esophagus inferiorly	Pharyngeal plexus	Narrows pharynx during swallowing
4. Palatopharyngeus	Soft palate	Thyroid cartilage, pharyngeal aponeurosis	Pharyngeal plexus	Narrows oropharyngeal opening, closes nasopharynx
5. Salpingopharyngeus	Auditory tube	Blends with palatopharyngeus	Pharyngeal plexus	Helps elevate nasopharynx
6. Stylopharyngeus	Base of styloid proc.	Thyroid cartilage and side of pharynx	Glossopharyngeal (IX)	Elevates and dilates pharynx

STUDY EXERCISES

1. Name the four muscles of mastication. By which cranial nerve are they innervated?

2. Which muscles are responsible for the grinding motion of the jaw during chewing? *Describe the origins and insertions of these muscles and how their attachments make the rotary motion possible.*

3. *Describe the attachments of the temporalis muscle and how its attachments relate to the actions of elevating and retracting the mandible.*

4. Name the most powerful elevator of the mandible.

5. Name the four infrahyoid muscles. Give their innervation and collective actions. *Give the origin and insertion for each muscle.*

6. Repeat Question 5 for the suprahyoid muscles.

7. Name the four extrinsic muscles of the tongue. Give their actions and innervation.

8. The muscles of facial expression are all innervated by what cranial nerve?

9. Name one muscle of facial expression for each of the following actions:

   A. Closes the eye
   B. Forms the substance of the cheek
   C. Wrinkles the skin of the forehead
   D. Closes the lips
   E. Raises the angle of the mouth
   F. Depresses the lower lip

10. Look in a mirror and smile. List the muscles involved in smiling as observed in the mirror. Now frown. Again, list the muscles that you observe as being necessary to produce the frown. It takes fewer muscles to smile than to frown. Conserve energy. Smile!

11. Name the three pharyngeal constrictor muscles. Name their common insertion, innervation, and action. *Describe their separate origins.*

12. *Name the three small muscles of the pharynx, and describe how they aid the constrictors during swallowing.*

13. Why are the muscles of the soft palate important during swallowing? Name the three muscles of the soft palate.

14. *Briefly describe the process of deglutition.*

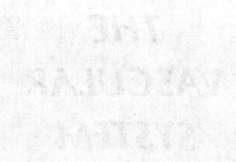

4

THE
VASCULAR
SYSTEM

LEARNING OBJECTIVES

At the conclusion of this chapter, the student should be able to:

1. Understand the origins of the arteries of the head and neck.
2. Diagram the branches of the external and internal carotid arteries and describe, in general terms, the areas supplied by these branches.
3. Describe the course, branches, and connections of the vertebral arteries.
4. Describe the Circle of Willis.
5. Appreciate the importance of the Circle of Willis and the many anastomoses of major vessels in the head and neck.
6. Give the names of, and areas drained by, the veins of the superficial and deep face.
7. Give the names, locations, and routes of drainage of the dural sinuses.
8. *Appreciate the interconnections of the veins and sinuses of the head and neck and their consequence for the spread of infection.*
9. Describe the components of the lymphatic system in the head and neck and their functions.
10. Be able to locate the various groups of nodes and describe the route of drainage of lymph from the head and neck.
11. Appreciate the significance of palpable lymph nodes.

The arteries begin at the heart and then branch out and diminish in size, becoming capillaries, which supply oxygen and nutrients to the tissues. The veins begin at the capillaries, increasing in size like streams feeding a river, until they reach the heart in the form of the superior and inferior vena cavae. Lymphatic vessels are similar to veins in pattern and function, ending in the venous system near the heart.

This pattern is somewhat modified in the head. Small veins that drain the brain empty into large dural sinuses, which empty into the jugular vein outside of the skull.

Anastomoses, or interconnections between blood vessels, are common throughout the circulatory system.

While the arteries, veins, and lymphatic system of the head and neck will be considered separately for convenience, it should be remembered that they function together, supplying nutrients and removing waste.

THE ARTERIES

The arteries supplying the head and neck are the carotid arteries and the vertebral arteries (Figure 4-1). The common carotid arteries arise, on the left, directly from the arch of the aorta and, on the right, from the brachiocephalic artery. Each common carotid ascends upward in the neck beneath the sternocleidomastoid muscle. At the upper margin of the thyroid cartilage, the common carotid bifurcates into internal and external branches. The internal branch enters the cranium through the carotid canal and supplies structures within. The external carotid supplies the head and neck outside the cranial cavity. The vertebral arteries arise from the right and left subclavian arteries near their origins. Each vertebral artery passes upward through the transverse foramina of the cervical vertebrae until it reaches the foramen magnum. The arteries enter the cranial cavity through the foramen magnum and, with the internal carotid artery, supply the structures within the cranial cavity.

External Carotid

The external carotid artery ascends in the neck to the level of the angle of the mandible (Figure 4-2). It is crossed by the posterior belly of the digastric and the stylohyoid muscles. Here the vessel ends, but its branches continue onto the face and scalp. The external carotid has eight branches: superior thyroid, ascending pharyngeal, lingual, facial, occipital, posterior auricular, superficial temporal, and maxillary.

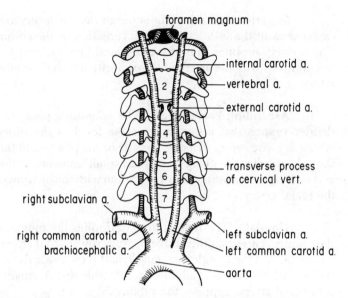

FIGURE 4–1 Origins of the arteries of the head and neck.

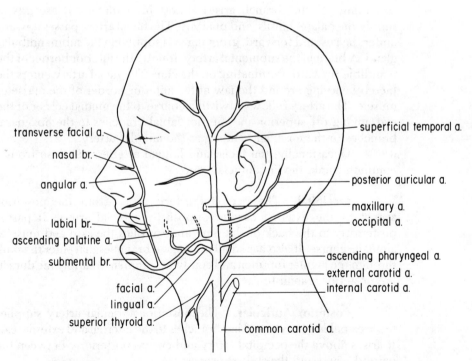

FIGURE 4–2 Origin and branches of the external carotid artery.

Superior Thyroid. The superior thyroid artery arises from the external carotid a little above the bifurcation of the common carotid. The artery supplies the thyroid gland and adjacent muscles. It anastomoses with the artery of the opposite side and the inferior thyroid artery.

Ascending Pharyngeal. The ascending pharyngeal is a very slender branch that arises at the same level as the superior thyroid artery. It passes upward along the side of the pharynx to the base of the skull. It supplies the pharynx and has small branches to the middle ear and meninges. Anastomoses are common with the pharyngeal branch of the facial artery.

Lingual. The lingual artery supplies the tongue and floor of the mouth. It arises a little above the superior thyroid artery. The artery passes behind the hyoglossus muscle and then upwards into the under-surface of the tongue all the way to the tip. A small branch, the sublingual artery, supplies the sublingual gland.

Facial. The facial artery arises superior to the lingual artery just below the angle of the jaw. It has a number of branches. The ascending palatine branch arises almost immediately. It ascends to supply the palate, tonsils, and pharynx. The facial artery passes upward under the jaw and forward, grooving and supplying the submandibular gland. A branch, the submental artery, follows the inferior border of the mandible forward, terminating on the chin. The facial artery enters the face by curving around the jaw at the anterior border of the masseter muscle. The artery follows a twisting course to the medial corner of the eye, giving off superior and inferior labial branches to the lips, nasal branches to the nose, and ending as the angular artery.

Occasionally, the facial and lingual arteries will arise from a common trunk, the linguofacial trunk.

Occipital. The occipital artery arises from the posterior aspect of the external carotid opposite the facial artery. It passes posteriorly to the back of the skull and supplies the skin and muscles along its course. It also has small meningeal branches that enter the skull through the jugular foramen and condylar foramen to supply the dura in the posterior cranial fossa.

Posterior Auricular. The posterior auricular artery supplies the area behind the ear and has branches to the internal and external ear. It arises above the occipital artery and curves posteriorly between the parotid gland and the styloid process.

Superficial Temporal. The terminal branches of the external carotid artery are the maxillary and superficial temporal arteries. The superficial temporal is the smaller of the two. It ascends deep to the parotid gland just in front of the ear. It gives off auricular branches to the ear and glandular branches to the parotid gland. Just before the superficial temporal emerges from the superior margin of the parotid gland, it gives off the transverse facial artery. This vessel passes horizontally across the face and anastomoses with the other facial vessels. Finally, the superficial temporal enters the temporal region and divides into anterior and posterior branches that supply the temporal and frontal regions.

Maxillary. The maxillary artery passes behind the head of the mandible, across the pterygoid muscles, and into the pterygopalatine fossa (Figure 4-3). It supplies the deep face and has a number of important branches. The middle meningeal artery is given off almost immediately. It passes upward, through the foramen spinosum, and into the cranial cavity to supply the meninges. The inferior alveolar artery passes downward from the maxillary artery and enters the mandibular canal to supply the teeth. The artery emerges through the mental foramen onto the chin and ends as the mental artery. The maxillary

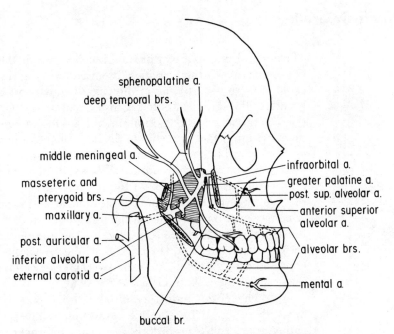

FIGURE 4-3   Origin and branches of the maxillary artery.

artery gives off muscular branches that may vary in number and origin. They are the deep temporal, pterygoid, masseteric, and buccal branches.

Near the pterygopalatine fossa, the posterior superior alveolar artery is given off. It descends along the back of the maxilla and divides into branches that enter the alveolar canals and supply the teeth, gums, and maxillary sinus. The infraorbital artery arises near the fossa and enters the orbit through the inferior orbital fissure. It then traverses the floor of the orbit in the infraorbital groove or canal and exits onto the face through the infraorbital foramen. It gives off orbital branches to structures in the orbit and anterior superior alveolar branches that supply the incisor and canine teeth and communicate with the posterior superior artery.

The greater palatine artery exits the pterygopalatine fossa through the greater palatine canal. It gives off the lesser palatine arteries and emerges onto the palate through the greater and lesser palatine foramina. They supply the palate.

The sphenopalatine artery is the terminal branch of the maxillary artery. It passes from the pterygopalatine fossa through the sphenopalatine foramen into the nose. Here it contributes to the vasculature of the nasal area.

Internal Carotid

The internal carotid artery has no branches outside the skull. It supplies the cranial and orbital cavities. It enters the skull through the carotid canal (Figure 4-4). While in the canal, it gives off a small tympanic branch to the ear. Upon entering the cranial cavity, the artery lies next to the sella turcica in a small dural sinus called the cavernous sinus. Here it gives off important branches to the hypophysis or pituitary gland. The internal carotid terminates in a number of branches. The ophthalmic artery arises from the carotid as it exits the cavernous sinus. The ophthalmic artery enters the orbit through the optic canal and supplies the eye. It terminates as the supratrochlear and supraorbital arteries, which emerge onto the face at the upper medial corner of the eye and the supraorbital foramen respectively. An anterior cerebral artery runs forward from the carotid to the frontal lobes. A small artery, the anterior communicating branch, joins the two anterior cerebral arteries across the front of the sella turcica.

The large middle cerebral arteries pass laterally and then upwards to supply the cerebral hemispheres. The posterior communicating arteries pass posteriorly from each internal carotid and join the

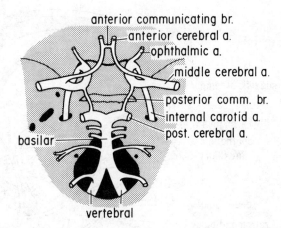

FIGURE 4–4   Branches of the internal carotid artery and the Circle of Willis.

posterior cerebral arteries. The vertebral arteries enter the cranial cavity through the foramen magnum as previously described. They immediately unite to form the basilar artery. The posterior cerebral arteries are terminal branches of the basilar artery. The union of the internal carotid arteries and posterior cerebral arteries through the posterior communicating arteries forms a ring of blood vessels called the *Circle of Willis* around the base of the brain. This arrangement provides a means for continued circulation to the brain should one of the carotid vessels be interrupted.

VEINS OF THE HEAD AND NECK

For purposes of description, the veins of the head and neck may be divided into two groups, those outside the cranial cavity and those inside the cranial cavity. However, it will become clear that there are many communications between the extra- and intracranial venous channels.

Veins of the External Head and Neck

The veins of the face and neck form a network of interconnected vessels that ends in the brachiocephalic and subclavian veins (Figure 4–5). Only the major vessels are described. Many variations exist in the pattern described here. However, the following is the most common.

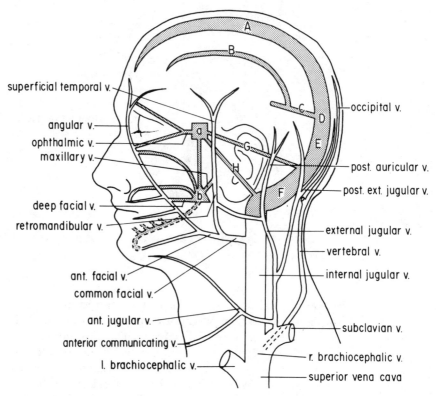

superficial temporal v.

angular v.
ophthalmic v.
maxillary v.

deep facial v.
retromandibular v.

ant. facial v.
common facial v.

ant. jugular v.
anterior communicating v.
l. brachiocephalic v.

occipital v.

post. auricular v.
post. ext. jugular v.

external jugular v.
vertebral v.
internal jugular v.

subclavian v.

r. brachiocephalic v.
superior vena cava

FIGURE 4–5   Veins and dural sinuses of the head and neck: (A) superior sagittal sinus, (B) inferior sagittal sinus, (C) straight sinus, (D) confluens sinuum, (E) transverse sinus, (F) sigmoid sinus, (G) superior petrosal sinus, (H) inferior petrosal sinus; (a) cavernous sinus, (b) pterygoid plexus. Stippled structures are deep.

Veins Draining the Superficial Face.   Blood from the superficial face is drained by the facial and superficial temporal veins. The facial vein drains the area supplied by the facial artery. The contributing veins are named like the arteries. The supraorbital and supratrochlear veins drain the region of the forehead supplied by the arteries of the same names. The veins unite at the medial corner of the eye to form the angular vein. The angular vein, like the angular artery, courses diagonally across the face. It is called the facial vein below its junction with the superior labial vein of the upper lip. The facial vein continues toward the anterior margin of the masseter muscle, where the facial artery enters the face. Here the facial vein curves under the inferior margin of the mandible and continues backward along it to the angle of the jaw.

The facial vein receives many branches along its course. It drains blood from the eyes, nose, lips, cheeks, and parotid gland. Below the mandible, it receives submandibular, submental, and tonsillar branches.

The superficial temporal vein begins over the temporal region. It drains portions of the scalp, ear, and parotid gland. It receives the transverse facial vein, which drains the zygomatic and lateral orbital regions. The superficial temporal vein is joined by the maxillary vein just in front of the earlobe to form the retromandibular vein. The retromandibular vein then divides into anterior and posterior branches. The anterior branch joins the facial vein at the angle of the jaw. The vein formed by this union is sometimes called the common facial vein. The common facial vein ends in the large, internal jugular vein. The internal jugular vein joins with the subclavian vein from the arm to form the brachiocephalic vein. The right and left brachiocephalic veins unite to form the superior vena cava, which empties into the heart.

Veins of the Deep Face

The Pterygoid Plexus.   Much of the venous blood from the deep face drains into the pterygoid plexus. The plexus is a collection of veins between the medial and lateral pterygoid muscles and the insertion of the temporalis muscle. Many branches from deep structures drain into the plexus. These include muscular branches from the temporalis, masseter, buccinator, and pterygoid muscles; sphenopalatine and palatine branches from the nose and palate; middle meningeal branches from the dura; and alveolar branches from the teeth. The pterygoid plexus and the facial vein are connected at the middle of the anterior margin of the masseter muscle by the deep facial vein. The plexus is drained by the maxillary vein, which joins the superficial temporal vein to form the retromandibular vein, as previously described.

Veins of the Teeth.   Blood from the mandibular teeth and gingiva is collected by interdental veins or a network of veins, the periapical plexus, which surrounds the apex of each tooth. Drainage proceeds into several inferior alveolar veins located in the mandibular canal. The alveolar veins from the anterior teeth join the facial vein through mental branches. Those from the posterior teeth drain into the pterygoid plexus. Blood from the maxillary teeth flows into the maxillary interdental or periapical plexus and then into veins accompanying the superior alveolar arteries. These vessels either join the facial vein anteriorly or the pterygoid plexus posteriorly.

Veins of the Tongue. The venous drainage of the tongue takes two courses. The blood from the dorsum and sides of the tongue drains into the lingual vein that accompanies the lingual artery and ends in the internal jugular vein. A second vein, the deep lingual, begins at the tip of the tongue on its undersurface. The vein joins the sublingual vein from the sublingual salivary gland at the anterior edge of the hyoglossus muscle. The new vein follows the hypoglossal nerve posteriorly and ends by joining the facial, internal jugular, or lingual vein.

Veins of the Posterior Scalp and Neck. Blood from the posterior region of the scalp is drained by the occipital vein, the posterior external jugular vein, and the external jugular vein. The external jugular vein is formed by the union of the posterior branch of the retromandibular vein and the posterior auricular vein. The posterior external jugular vein receives blood from the posterolateral scalp. It joins the external jugular at its midpoint. The external jugular then descends and ends in the subclavian vein. The occipital vein begins high on the back of the scalp. It passes deep beneath the trapezius muscle to join the vertebral vein at its origin near the base of the skull. The vertebral vein descends in the neck through the transverse foramina of the cervical vertebrae and ends in the back of the brachiocephalic vein near its origin.

Venous blood of the anterior neck region is drained by the anterior jugular vein. It begins near the hyoid bone, draining blood from the suprahyoid region. It is joined by tributaries from the thyroid gland and larynx. The vein descends diagonally and ends in the external jugular vein near its termination in the subclavian vein. While there are usually two anterior jugular veins, a right and a left, it is not uncommon to find a single vein located down the midline of the neck. When two vessels are present, they are usually joined by a large communicating branch, the jugular arch, at the base of the neck just above the sternum. The jugular arch may receive one or more inferior thyroid veins.

Veins of the Cranial Cavity, the Dural Sinuses

There are many named veins that drain the brain and meninges. Most of them, however, drain into the large dural sinuses, all of which eventually empty into the internal jugular vein.

In order to understand the dural sinuses, it is necessary to describe the dura.

The Dura Mater. The dura mater is a tough membrane that lines the cranial cavity and spinal canal and supports the brain (Figure 4–6). It is very closely opposed to the interior of the cranium. The dura consists of two layers that are held tightly together except at certain places which house the dural venous sinuses. The dura projects into the cranial cavity as a series of septa that divide the cavity into spaces which house subdivisions of the brain.

Falx Cerebri.   The falx cerebri is a septum of dura that projects vertically in the sagittal plane between the two cerebral hemispheres. It is attached to the crista galli anteriorly and the tentorium cerebelli posteriorly.

Tentorium Cerebelli.   The tentorium cerebelli is a shelf of dura that separates the occipital lobes of the brain from the cerebellum. It is attached to the occipital bone along the groove for the transverse sinus. Each side projects laterally and forward, encircling the base and the midbrain; attaches to the top of the petrous temporal bone; and ends at the anterior clinoid processes.

Falx Cerebelli.   A small dural septum projecting between the lobes of the cerebellum is called the falx cerebelli.

Diaphragma Sellae.   The dura covering the sella turcica is called the diaphragma sellae. It is perforated by the stalk of the pituitary gland, which attaches the gland beneath the diaphragma to the brain above it.

The dural sinuses are venous spaces located between the layers of dura mater (Figure 4–5).

The Dural Sinuses.   The superior sagittal sinus lies at the attached margin of the falx cerebri. It begins at the crista galli and grooves the parietal bones along the sagittal suture and the occipital bone to the internal occipital protuberance. The inferior sagittal sinus is located in the inferior free margin of the falx cerebri. It is connected to the superior sinus by the straight sinus, which occupies the junction of the falx cerebri and tentorium cerebelli. The transverse sinuses curve laterally from the superior sagittal sinus at the internal occipital protuberance. They groove the occipital bone transversely along the attachment of the tentorium cerebelli. Upon reaching the posterolateral end of the petrous temporal bone, the transverse sinus becomes the sigmoid sinus as it cuts a deep "S"-shaped groove, ending at the jugular foramen. The occipital sinus is located in the attached margin of the falx cerebelli and empties into the junction of the straight, superior sagittal, and transverse sinuses at the internal occipital protuberance. This area of union of the sinuses is called the sinus confluens.

The cavernous sinuses lie in the dura on each side of the sella turcica. The sinuses communicate with each other across the sella anteriorly and posteriorly. The cavernous sinuses receive the ophthalmic veins from the orbits and communicate with the pterygoid plexus.

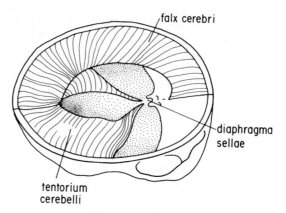

FIGURE 4–6   Cranial dura.

They drain posteriorly via the superior and inferior petrosal sinuses. The superior petrosal sinus lies in the tentorium cerebelli along the top of the petrous temporal bone and ends in the transverse sinus. The inferior petrosal sinus drains the cavernous sinus into the origin of the internal jugular vein at the jugular foramen. It lies in the dura and a groove between the petrous temporal bone and the basilar part of the occipital bone.

All of the venous blood of the cranial cavity drains into the internal jugular vein.

The veins and sinuses described above communicate with whatever veins are nearby. In addition, small vessels called emissary veins connect the interior and exterior venous systems. The extensive interconnections of the intra- and extracranial venous systems have several consequences. Should one of the internal jugular veins become occluded, the intracranial pressure would increase due to damming of blood within the rigid cranial vault. However, this pressure can be reduced by shunting blood from the sinuses to the exterior through the ophthalmic veins, pterygoid plexus, or many diploic or emissary veins. Thus, the alternate circulatory pathways act as a safety valve. Also, because the veins and sinuses have no valves, blood may flow in either direction. It is possible for extracranial infections to be carried into the cranial cavity.

LYMPHATIC SYSTEM OF THE HEAD AND NECK

Lymph is a clear, colorless, slightly alkaline fluid found in lymphatic vessels. It is formed in tissue spaces all over the body and is much like blood plasma. The exact composition of lymph differs depending on the part of the body from which it is collected. It is composed mostly of extravascular water, protein, and particulate material (including bacteria). The cells found in lymph are primarily lymphocytes.

The lymphatic system of the head and neck consists of lymph vessels, lymph nodes, tonsils, and thymus. The lymphatic system serves two functions: (1) it helps the venous system transport fluid from the tissues back into the circulation; and (2) it forms a part of the body's defense system. If the lymphatic system fails to function and the flow of lymph is interrupted, fluid will accumulate in the tissues resulting in a swollen, puffy appearance. This condition is called *edema*.

Lymph Vessels

Lymph vessels begin in the tissue spaces as capillaries. They drain away fluid, protein, and particulate matter not removed by the veins. The capillaries join to form larger vessels. The vessels are thinner and more delicate than veins. Lymph from the right arm, right side of the torso, and right side of the head and neck eventually empties into the right lymphatic duct, which, in turn, ends in the right subclavian vein. The lymph from the rest of the body flows into a lymph vessel called the thoracic duct, which empties into the left subclavian vein.

Lymph Nodes

Lymph nodes are small, bean-shaped organs along the course of lymph vessels. Nodes may occur singly or in groups and vary in size. They contain macrophages that remove particulate matter, especially bacteria, from the lymph before it is returned to the blood. The vessel that brings lymph into the node is called *afferent*, and the vessel that carries lymph away from the node is called *efferent*. Each node has several afferent vessels and usually a single efferent vessel. Nodes also contain lymphoid cells, which reproduce when stimulated to do so by infection. Resting nodes are usually small and not readily palpable. Stimulated nodes become swollen with new cells and tender to the touch. Swollen nodes indicate the presence of a pathologic condition. Knowledge of the location of lymph nodes and the areas drained by the afferent vessels of each node aids in diagnosing the location of the pathology.

Lymphatic Drainage of the Head and Neck

Deep Cervical Nodes.   The lymph nodes of the head and neck are divided into superficial groups and deep groups (Figure 4-7). The deep cervical nodes and vessels connecting them are located along the course of the internal jugular vein. They may be divided into a superior and an inferior group according to their location along the vein. All of the lymph from the head and face eventually drains into these nodes and then into the thoracic duct or right lymphatic duct.

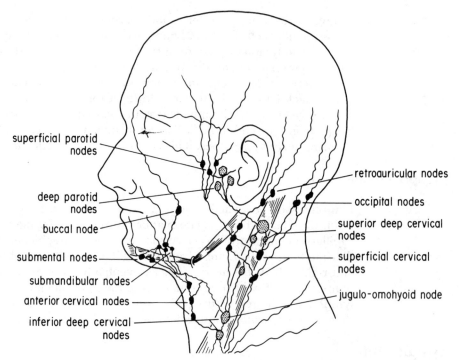

superficial parotid
nodes

retroauricular nodes

deep parotid
nodes

occipital nodes

buccal node

superior deep cervical
nodes

submental nodes

superficial cervical
nodes

submandibular nodes

anterior cervical nodes

jugulo-omohyoid node

inferior deep cervical
nodes

FIGURE 4–7   Lymph nodes and vessels of the head and neck.

The superior deep cervical nodes are located at the upper end of the jugular vein beneath the sternocleidomastoid muscle. Some nodes from this group are located at the medial border of the sterno-cleidomastoid between it and the digastric muscle.

The inferior deep cervical group is found beneath the sterno-cleidomastoid muscle on the lower portion of the internal jugular vein. It receives lymph from the upper deep cervical nodes through a large vessel, the jugular trunk. One large node of this group is located just above the intermediate tendon of the omohyoid. It is called the jugulo-omohyoid node and receives much of the lymph from the tongue. The jugular trunk usually joins the right lymphatic duct or thoracic duct on the left side, but the jugular trunk may empty directly into the ipsilateral subclavian vein.

Groups of nodes flank the trachea, esophagus, larynx, pharynx, and thyroid gland. They receive lymph from these structures and pass it along to the deep cervical nodes.

Superficial Lymph Nodes.   The superficial lymph nodes are named by their location. The most constant nodes are the parotid, posterior, auricular, occipital, buccal, submandibular, submental, anterior cervical, and superficial cervical groups.

The superficial parotid nodes are located under the fascia of the parotid gland. They receive afferent lymph vessels from the temporal, zygomatic, and lateral eye regions and the anterior part of the ear. Efferent vessels from the parotid nodes drain into the superior deep cervical nodes. Deep parotid nodes are located in the substance of the parotid gland. They receive lymph from the middle ear, eyelids, and conjunctiva. These nodes also drain into the superior deep cervical nodes.

The posterior auricular lymph nodes receive lymph from the skin and scalp behind and above the ear and from the posterior part of the external ear. They are located in the connective tissues over the mastoid process. The occipital nodes are located at the attachment of the trapezius muscle to the skull. They drain lymph from the occipital region. Efferent vessels from the posterior auricular and occipital nodes empty into the superior deep cervical nodes.

Lymph from the nose, cheek, upper lip, lateral part of the lower lip, teeth, gums, and anterior hard palate drains into the submandibular lymph nodes. Afferent vessels follow the course of the facial vein. A buccal node is usually located in the buccal fascia along the course of these vessels. The submandibular nodes lie on the mylohyoid muscle between the anterior belly of the digastric muscle and the mandible. The central part of the lower lip, the chin, the floor of the mouth, and the tongue are drained by lymph vessels, which are afferents to the submental lymph nodes. These nodes lie on the mylohyoid muscle between the anterior bellies of the digastric muscles. Lymph from the submental nodes flows into the submandibular nodes or directly into the jugulo-omohyoid node of the inferior deep cervical group.

All of the lymph from the face and scalp drains into the deep cervical nodes. However, one other group, the superficial cervical nodes may intervene. The superficial cervical nodes lie on the surface of the sternocleidomastoid muscle along the course of the external jugular vein. These nodes receive some of the lymph from the angle of the jaw and ear. They are connected to the deep cervical nodes and drain into them.

One other group of superficial nodes, the anterior cervical nodes, lies along the course of the anterior jugular vein. These nodes receive lymph from the infrahyoid region. Like the other groups, they drain into the deep cervical nodes.

Table 4-1 summarizes the groups of nodes draining specific areas. While the exact pattern of drainage varies, the principal groups of nodes and vessels are constant enough to be of diagnostic use.

TABLE 4–1 Summary of Routes of Lymphatic Drainage

Nodes	Receive Lymph From	Drain Into
Superficial parotid nodes	Temporal, zygomatic, and lateral eye region and anterior ear	Superior deep cervical nodes
Deep parotid nodes	Middle ear, eyelids, and conjunctiva	Superior deep cervical nodes
Posterior auricular nodes	Skin and scalp behind and above the ear, posterior external ear	Superior deep cervical nodes
Occipital nodes	Occipital region	Superior deep cervical nodes
Submandibular nodes	Nose and paranasal sinuses, cheek, upper lip, lateral lower lip, teeth, gingiva, anterior hard palate, lymph from submental nodes	Superior and inferior deep cervical nodes
Submental nodes	Central lower lip, chin, floor of mouth, tongue	Submandibular nodes of jugulo-omohyoid node of the inferior deep cervical nodes
Superficial cervical nodes	Angle of the jaw and ear	Deep cervical nodes
Anterior cervical nodes	Infrahyoid region	Deep cervical nodes
Deep cervical nodes	Face and scalp directly, all other groups indirectly	Right lymphatic duct or thoracic duct

Other Lymphatic Organs

Tonsils.   Tonsils are collections of lymphoid tissue that are thought to function as defense organs. They do not filter lymph and are not supplied with lymph vessels. There are three major tonsils: the palatine, the pharyngeal, and the sublingual. They will be discussed in conjunction with the oral cavity.

Thymus.   The thymus gland is of supreme importance to the proper functioning of the immune system. It is located at the base of the neck in the thoracic cavity and overlies a portion of the heart and great vessels. It is large in the newborn and at puberty but regresses in later life. Congenital absence leads to overwhelming infections and death. The thymus gland is the subject of extensive research and is beyond the scope of this text.

CHAPTER SUMMARY

Arteries of the Head and Neck

Main Artery	Major Branch	Secondary Branches	Area Supplied
External carotid	1. Superior thyroid		Thyroid gland
	2. Ascending pharyngeal		Pharynx, middle ear, meninges
	3. Lingual		Tongue and floor of mouth
	4. Facial	1. Ascending palatine	Palate, tonsils, pharynx
		2. Submental	Skin and muscles of chin
		3. Labial	Lips
		4. Nasal	Nose
		5. Angular	Terminal branch ending at the medial corner of the eye
	5. Occipital		Back of the skull, muscles, and scalp
	6. Posterior auricular		Skin and muscles behind the ear; internal and external ear
	7. Superficial temporal	1. Auricular br.	Ear
		2. Glandular	Parotid gland
		3. Transverse facial	Middle of the face
		4. Anterior temporal	Frontal region
		5. Posterior temporal	Temporal region
	8. Maxillary	1. Middle meningeal	Meninges
		2. Inferior alveolar	Mandibular teeth, ends at the mental a. on the chin
		3. Muscular branches	Temporalis, Masseter, Buccinator, Pterygoids
		4. Posterior superior alveolar	Maxillary teeth, gingiva, maxillary sinus
		5. Infraorbital	Skin and muscles of the mid face
		a. Anterior superior alveolar	Maxillary canine and incisor teeth
		b. Orbital branches	Orbit
		6. Greater palatine	Palate
		7. Sphenopalatine	Nose
Internal carotid	1. Tympanic br.		Ear
	2. Hypophyseal brs.		Pituitary gland

Arteries of the Head and Neck (continued)

Main Artery	Major Branch	Secondary Branches	Area Supplied
	3. Ophthalmic	1. Supratrochlear	Eye, skin, and muscles of the supraorbital and frontal region
		2. Supraorbital	
	4. Anterior cerebral		Frontal lobes of brain
		Anterior communicating br.	Joins the anterior cerebrals in front of the sella turcica
	5. Middle cerebral		Cerebral hemispheres
	6. Posterior communi- cating br.		Joins the posterior cerebrals
Vertebral	Join to form the basilar	Posterior cerebrals	The cerebral hemispheres. Together with the branches of the internal carotid, they form the Circle of Willis

Veins of the Head and Neck

Area Drained	Veins	Contributing Brs.	Major Vessel of Drainage
Superficial face	Facial vein	1. Supraorbital 2. Supratrochlear 3. Angular 4. Labial 5. Mental	Retromandibular v. union of facial and retromandibular forms common facial v.
	Common facial v.		
Temporal region	Superficial temporal	Transverse facial	Joins the maxillary v. to form the retromandibular
Scalp, ear, parotid gland	Retro- mandibular v.	1. Anterior br.	Joins the facial v. to form the common facial v.
		2. Posterior br.	Joins the external jugular v.
Posterior scalp and neck	1. posterior auricular		Joins the posterior br. of the retromandibular to form the external jugular v.
	2. Posterior external jugular		Joins the external jugular
	3. External jugular		Joins the subclavian v.
	4. Occipital v.		Joins the vertebral
	5. Vertebral		Joins the brachiocephalic v.
Anterior neck	Anterior jugular v.	1. Suprahyoid vs.	The anterior jugular joins the external jugular v.

Veins of the Head and Neck (continued)

Area Drained	Veins	Contributing Brs.	Major Vessel of Drainage
		2. Thyroid vs.	
		3. Laryngeal vs.	
		4. Communicating br.	Joins the anterior jugular vs. at the base of the neck
Deep face	1. Pterygoid plexus	1. Muscular brs. from temporalis, masseter, buccinator, pterygoids	The pterygoid plexus is drained by the maxillary v.
		2. Sphenopalatine and palatine brs. from the nose and palate	
		3. Middle meningeal brs. from dura	
		4. Alveolar brs. from the teeth	
	2. Deep facial v.		Connects the facial vein and pterygoid plexus
	3. Maxillary v.		Drains the pterygoid plexus, joins the superficial temporal to form the retromandibular v.
Mandibular teeth	Inferior alveolar vs.	Interdental veins or periapical plexus	Pterygoid plexus
Maxillary teeth	Superior alveolar vs.	Interdental veins or periapical plexus	Pterygoid plexus or facial v.
Tongue	1. Lingual v.		Internal jugular v.
	2. Deep lingual v.		Joins the sublingual v. and ends in the facial, internal jugular, or lingual v.

Dural Sinuses

Sinus	Receives Blood From	Location	Drains Into
Superior sagittal	Brain and dura	Superior edge of falx cerebri	Sinus confluens
Inferior sagittal	Brain and dura	Inferior edge of falx cerebri	Straight sinus
Straight sinus	Inferior sagittal	Junction of falx cerebri and tentorium cerebelli	Sigmoid sinus

Dural Sinuses (continued)

Sinus	Receives Blood From	Location	Drains Into
Sigmoid sinus	*Transverse sinus*	Posterolateral end of petrous temporal bone	*Internal jugular v.*
Occipital sinus	*Occipital region*	Attached margin of falx cerebelli	*Sinus confluens*
Cavernous sinuses	*Superior and inferior ophthalmic vs., pterygoid plexus*	Either side of sella turcica	*Sup. and inf. petrosal sinuses*
Superior petrosal sinus	*Cavernous sinus*	Tentorium cerebelli along top of petrous temporal bone	*Transverse sinus*
Inferior petrosal sinus	*Cavernous sinus*	In dura at junction of petrous temporal bone and basilar part of occipital bone	*Origin of internal jugular v.*

STUDY EXERCISES

1. Diagram the origins of the common carotid arteries from the aortic arch.
2. Diagram the branches of the external carotid artery to the superficial face.
3. *Diagram the branches of the maxillary artery.*
4. Name the vessels that blood would flow through to get to each of the following structures. More than one route is possible in some cases.

   A. Maxillary molar teeth
   B. Tongue
   C. Palate
   D. Chin
   E. Palatine tonsil
   F. Muscles of mastication
   G. Skin of the temporal region
   H. Mandibular teeth
   I. Maxillary sinus

5. *Diagram the Circle of Willis.*
6. *If the right common carotid artery were to become blocked, how would blood get to the right side of the brain? To the right lingual artery? To the right occipital artery?*
7. Name the veins through which blood being drained from the following regions would flow.

   A. Eye
   B. Tongue
   C. Maxillary teeth
   D. Superior sagittal sinus
   E. Parotid gland
   F. Suprahyoid muscles

8. Explain how bacteria from an infected molar tooth could spread into the cranial cavity.
9. State two functions of lymph nodes.
10. Which nodes receive lymph from each of the following areas?

    A. Nose and paranasal sinuses
    B. Angle of the jaw and ear
    C. Zygomatic region
    D. Teeth
    E. Floor of the mouth
    F. Infrahyoid region
    G. Tongue

5

THE
NERVOUS
SYSTEM

LEARNING OBJECTIVES

At the conclusion of this chapter, the student should be able to:

1. Recognize and describe a cross-section of the cervical spinal cord and spinal nerve.
2. *Describe briefly the distribution of the dorsal rami of the cervical spinal nerves.*
3. *Describe briefly the distribution of the ventral rami of the cervical spinal nerves and the cervical plexus.*
4. *Name the major parts and divisions of the brain.*
5. Give the names and numbers of the cranial nerves.
6. Be able to state the components (sensory and/or motor), ganglia, distribution, and function of the fifth and seventh cranial nerves.
7. *Summarize the components, ganglia, distribution, and function of the cranial nerves.*
8. Appreciate the similarities and differences between the sympathetic and parasympathetic nervous systems.
9. Briefly describe the sympathetic nervous system in the head and neck including ganglia, distribution, and function.
10. Briefly describe the parasympathetic nervous system in the head and neck including preganglionic nerve, postganglionic nerve, ganglion, distribution, and function.

The functional unit of the nervous system is the nerve cell or neuron. The neuron consists of a nerve cell body and extensions of it called *nerve fibers*. There are two types of fibers: dendrites, which bring information to the nerve cell; and axons, which carry information away from the cell body. A nerve cell may have many dendrites, but it usually has just one axon. The dendrites usually arise from the cell body and project outward like fingers. The axon arises from an area of the cell body called the axon hillock but it may arise from the base of one of the dendrites. Both types of fibers vary in length. A cell with many dendrites and one axon is called multipolar. This is typical of motor neurons. A cell with a single dendrite and one axon arising from opposite poles is called bipolar. Bipolar cells are found in the retina and other organs of special sense. A neuron with a single fiber that divides into a dendrite and an axon is called unipolar. Sensory nerve cells are typically unipolar.

Nerve fibers may be insulated with a material called myelin. Myelin results from repeated wrapping of the fiber by specialized cells. Outside the central nervous system, these cells are called Schwann cells. Inside the brain and spinal cord, this function is performed by non-neuronal cells called glial cells. Myelin sheaths give the fibers a glistening, white appearance.

The brain and spinal cord are called the central nervous system (CNS). The peripheral nervous system includes the cranial nerves and spinal nerves along with their branches and ganglia. A ganglion is a collection of nerve cells outside the CNS.

THE CERVICAL SPINAL CORD

The spinal cord is the continuation of the brain into the vertebral canal. It may be divided into cervical, thoracic, lumbar, and sacral regions. In cross section, the different regions vary significantly. However, some general characteristics prevail. The center of the spinal cord presents a grayish butterfly-shaped area, the gray matter (Figure 5–1). This area consists of nerve cell bodies arranged in functional groups. The posterior projections of the gray matter are called the dorsal gray columns, and the anterior projection is called the ventral gray columns. The cells in the dorsal columns are sensory in function, while those in the ventral columns are motor cells.

The gray matter is perforated in the center by the central canal and is surrounded on the outside by the white matter. The white matter consists of mostly myelinated fibers from nerve cells both inside and outside the spinal cord. These fibers run up and down the spinal cord making contact with neurons in the brain and other levels of the cord. The fibers are functionally grouped and make up fiber tracts within the cord.

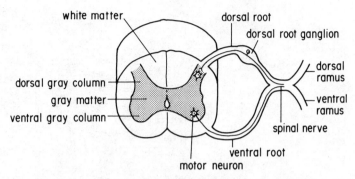

FIGURE 5–1   Cross-section of the spinal cord.

Fibers from motor neurons of the ventral gray column emerge from the cord at regular intervals and are called ventral spinal roots. Sensory fibers enter the cord on its dorso-lateral aspect to make contact with cells in the dorsal gray column. These fibers constitute the dorsal spinal roots. Outside of the spinal cord, the cell bodies from which the fibers of the dorsal spinal roots arise are located in ganglia called dorsal root ganglia. The neurons of the dorsal root ganglia are unipolar. One end of the fiber from each neuron leaves one side of the ganglion and enters the spinal cord, forming the dorsal root. The other end of the fiber of each neuron exits the opposite side of the ganglion and joins with the ventral root to form a spinal nerve. The spinal nerve exits the vertebral canal through the intervertebral foramen. The first cervical spinal nerve is an exception. It passes between the atlas and occipital bone. There are eight cervical nerves, twelve thoracic nerves, five lumbar nerves, five sacral nerves and one coccygeal spinal nerve. They are commonly identified by the abbreviations C, T, L, S, and Co, followed by the appropriate number.

The Cervical Spinal Nerves

When the spinal nerves emerge from the intervertebral foramina, they divide into dorsal and ventral rami. Each ramus may consist of a mixture of motor and sensory fibers or it may be almost purely motor or purely sensory, depending upon its final destination.

Dorsal Rami of Cervical Spinal Nerves.   The dorsal rami of all cervical spinal nerves innervate the muscles of the suboccipital and posterior neck region. In addition, dorsal rami of C2, 3, 4, and 5 supply sensory innervation to the skin of this area.

Ventral Rami of Cervical Spinal Nerves.   The ventral rami of the cervical spinal nerves pass anteriorly. Those of C1, 2, 3, and 4 unite in

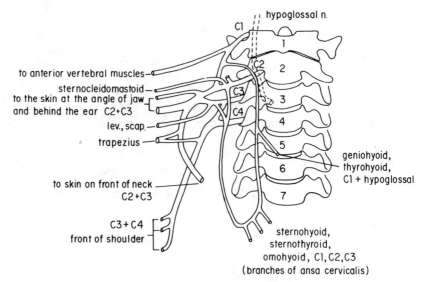

FIGURE 5–2   Diagram of the cervical plexus.

a meshwork of nerves called the cervical plexus (Figure 5–2). This plexus supplies motor innervation to the anterior vertebral muscles, lateral neck muscles, infrahyoid muscles, and geniohyoid and thyrohyoid muscles.

In addition, it supplies sensory innervation to the skin of the posterior scalp, posterior and inferior auricular region, posterolateral and lateral neck regions, anterior neck, and submandibular region. The ventral rami of C5, 6, 7, and 8 contribute to the brachial plexus which, along with T1, innervates the arm.

THE BRAIN AND CRANIAL NERVES

The portion of the head not supplied by the cervical spinal nerves is supplied by the cranial nerves. A brief description of the brain will aid in understanding the origins of the cranial nerves.

The Brain

The brain consists of the cerebral hemispheres, the cerebellar hemispheres, and the brain stem to which the cerebrum and cerebellum are attached (Figure 5–3). The cerebral hemispheres are separated from one another by a medial longitudinal fissure. At the bottom of this fissure, they are joined by a thick, elongated band of fibers, the corpus callosum (Figure 5–4). The cerebral hemispheres are attached to the

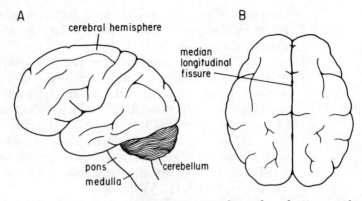

FIGURE 5-3   Views of the brain: (A) lateral and (B) superior.

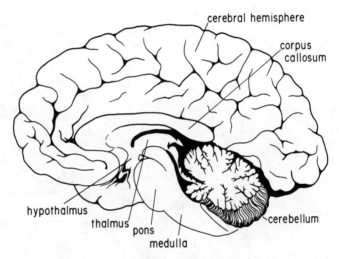

FIGURE 5-4   Sagittal section of the brain.

brain stem by thick fiber tracts, the cerebral peduncles. The surface of the cerebrum is highly convoluted, increasing the surface area considerably. Unlike the spinal cord, the gray matter or cells cover the surface and are called the cortex, while the fiber tracts occupy the center. The cortex is thought to be where the final integration of neural mechanisms takes place. It is considered to be the location of personality and intellect. In truth, we have only begun to understand the functions of the cerebral cortex.

The cerebellum is located beneath the posterior or occipital lobes of the cerebrum (Figure 5-5). Like the cerebrum, it consists of a cellular cortex over a fibrous center and is connected to the brain stem by cerebellar peduncles. The cerebellum coordinates the actions of muscles throughout the body.

The brain stem may be divided into the medulla, pons, midbrain, and diencephalon (Figure 5-4). The medulla is continuous with the spinal cord at the foramen magnum. It is made up of fiber tracts and collections of nerve cells called nuclei, which are the origins of some of the cranial nerves (VII, IX, X, XI, and XII).

The pons is a large, squarish mass anterior to, and continuous with, the medulla. The cerebral peduncles enter its superior surface. It, too, is composed of fiber tracts and nuclei, some of which give origin to cranial nerves III, IV, V, and VI.

The midbrain is a short section between the pons and the diencephalon. Its composition is similar to the pons and gives rise to portions of some of the same cranial nerves.

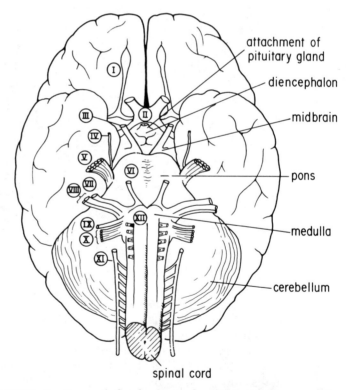

FIGURE 5-5   Base of the brain and origins of the cranial nerves: olfactory (I), optic (II), oculomotor (III), trochlear (IV), trigeminal (V), abducens (VI), facial (VII), vestibulocochlear (VIII), glossopharyngeal (IX), vagus (X), spinal accessory (XI), and hypoglossal (XII).

The diencephalon is a complex area anterior to the midbrain and beneath the cerebral hemispheres. It contains two very important areas: the thalamus and hypothalamus. The thalamus is a switching station for all kinds of information en route to the cerebral cortex. The hypothalamus produces hormones, some of which are stored in the posterior pituitary gland. Other hormones produced here act on the anterior pituitary, effecting the release of pituitary hormones. The hyopthalamus also contains centers for the control of appetite, body temperature, and emotions. The olfactory and optic nerves (cranial nerves I and II) have connections in the diencephalon.

The Cranial Nerves

There are twelve cranial nerves. They are numbered in the order in which they are attached to the brain, beginning at the anterior extreme with the olfactory nerve.

Some cranial nerves, like the optic nerve, are entirely sensory in function (Figure 5-4). Some are entirely motor, like the hypoglossal, which supplies innervation to the muscles of the tongue. Some cranial nerves are composed of both sensory and motor fibers, like the trigeminal nerve, which supplies sensory innervation to the face and motor innervation to the muscles of mastication.

As in the spinal nerves, the nerve cell bodies of motor and sensory neurons are located in different places. Nerve cell bodies of motor neurons are located in various areas called nuclei in the brain stem. Cell bodies of sensory neurons of cranial nerves are found in the sensory ganglia associated with that particular cranial nerve. Like the neurons of the dorsal root ganglia, the cells are unipolar and send one end of their fiber into the brain stem while the other end is distributed to the area to be innervated. The optic, olfactory, and vestibulocochlear nerves, however, are special sensory nerves. The cell bodies from which the fibers of these nerves arise are located in the retina of the eye, the olfactory epithelium of the nose, and the vestibular apparatus and cochlea of the ear respectively. The fibers of these nerves then form tracts which pass into the brain to be integrated and perceived.

The Olfactory Nerve (I).   The olfactory receptors make up the specialized epithelium of the nose and are located on the superior nasal concha and roof of the nasal cavities (Figure 5-6). The receptor cells send out fibers that pass through the fenestrated cribriform plate of the ethmoid bone. The olfactory bulbs lie on the intracranial surface of the cribriform plates. The fibers from the nasal epithelium constitute the olfactory nerves. These nerves enter the bulbs and synapse with cells there. Fibers from these cells form the olfactory tracts, which enter the

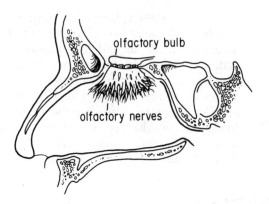

FIGURE 5–6   The olfactory nerve.

brain in front of the optic chiasma. The olfactory nerves are entirely sensory. Destruction of the olfactory epithelium, nerves, or tracts results in anosmia, loss of sense of smell, and consequently a loss of taste quality.

The Optic Nerve (II).   The optic nerve is formed from fibers of the neurons that make up the retina of the eye. The nerve exits from the orbit through the optic foramen. It meets its fellow from the opposite side and a portion of the fibers from each side cross to the other side of the optic chiasma just behind the anterior clinoid processes. The new collections of fibers are called the optic tracts. They enter the brain. Destruction of the retina or complete section of the optic nerve causes blindness in the affected eye. Complete section of the optic tract causes visual defects in both eyes.

The Oculomotor Nerve (III).   The oculomotor nerve provides the motor innervation to four of the six eye muscles that move the eyeball: the superior, inferior, and medial rectus muscles and the inferior oblique muscle (Figure 5-7). It also innervates the pupillary muscle, which contracts the pupil, and the ciliary muscle, whose contraction thickens the lens. It emerges from the brain just anterior to the pons between the cerebral preduncles (Figure 5-4). Damage causes deviation of the eyeball, squint, dilation of the pupil with loss of light reflexes, and loss of accommodation by the lens.

The Trochlear (IV) and Abducens (VI) Nerves.   The trochlear (IV) and abducens (VI) nerves provide motor innervation to the remaining two muscles of the eyeball. The trochlear nerve emerges from the brain stem on the dorsal surface and curves around the base of the cerebral peduncles to enter the orbit (Figure 5-7). It innervates the

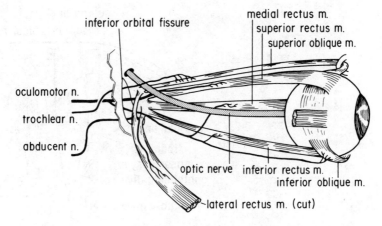

FIGURE 5–7 Cranial nerves to the muscles of the eye.

superior oblique muscle. The abducens nerve arises at the junction of the medulla and pons on the ventral surface. It innervates the lateral rectus muscle. Damage to these nerves results in deviation of the eyeball and inability to move the eyeball laterally.

The Trigeminal Nerve (V). The trigeminal nerve (V) is the largest cranial nerve. It provides sensory innervation to the face, scalp, nose, mouth, and teeth. A small motor component supplies the muscles of mastication. It is attached to the anterior inferior surface of the pons. The cells of the sensory portion, or root, are located in the large, semilunar ganglion that lies in a depression on the anterior superior surface of the petrous temporal bone. The fibers from these unipolar sensory neurons divide into central and peripheral branches. The central branches make up the sensory root. They pass from the posterior surface of the ganglion and enter the pons. The peripheral fibers exit the anterior edge of the ganglion in three separate divisions: the ophthalmic, the maxillary, and the mandibular. The small motor root of the trigeminal emerges from the brain where the sensory root enters. All of the motor fibers pass, unimpeded, through the semilunar ganglion and join with the mandibular division. The ophthalmic and maxillary divisions are purely sensory.

The Ophthalmic Nerve. The ophthalmic division of the trigeminal, or ophthalmic, nerve is the smallest division (Figure 5–8). It supplies sensory innervation to the orbit, lacrimal gland, nose, and skin of the eylids and forehead. The nerve enters the orbit through the superior orbital fissure and divides into lacrimal, frontal, and nasociliary branches. The lacrimal branch passes laterally and supplies the lacrimal

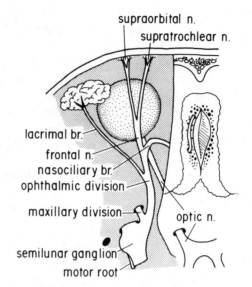

FIGURE 5–8   Ophthalmic division of the trigeminal nerve.

gland. It then pierces the skin and supplies the upper eyelid. The frontal nerve passes forward in the orbit and divides into supratrochlear and supraorbital branches.

The supratrochlear branch continues forward medially and passes out of the orbit between the supraorbital foramen and the nose. It supplies a portion of the skin of the forehead. The supraorbital nerve exits the orbit through the supraorbital foramen or notch and supplies the skin of the forehead and scalp.

The nasociliary nerve gives off sensory branches within the orbit and then pierces the medial wall of the orbit and enters the cranial cavity at the posterior end of the cribriform plate. It then runs forward on the plate and down into the nose through a slit at the side of the crista galli. It supplies the inside of the nose and then ends in the skin of the nose.

The tiny ciliary ganglion lies near the optic and nasociliary nerves. It is an autonomic ganglion and will be discussed with the autonomic nervous system.

The Maxillary Nerve.   The maxillary division of the trigeminal nerve is also purely sensory (Figures 5–9 and 5–10). Its branches supply the skin of the middle of the face, the upper lip, the nose and nasal mucosa, the maxillary teeth, the palatal gingiva, and the palate. After leaving the semilunar ganglion, the nerve exits the cranial cavity through the foramen rotundum and enters the pterygopalatine fossa. In the

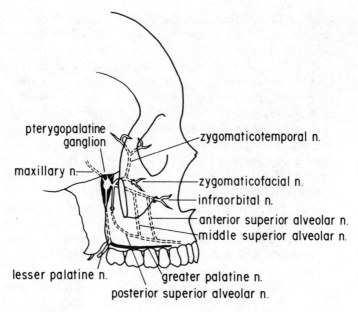

FIGURE 5-9   Maxillary division of the trigeminal nerve.

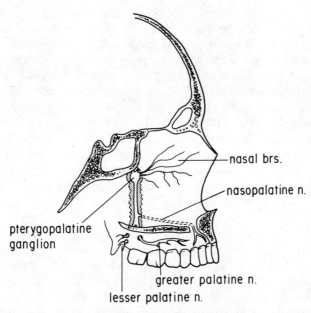

FIGURE 5-10   Maxillary division of the trigeminal nerve in the nose and palate.

pterygopalatine fossa, the maxillary nerve divides into four branches: the infraorbital, the zygomatic, the posterior superior alveolar, and the palatine. The infraorbital nerve passes forward and enters the posterior end of the infraorbital groove. It traverses the infraorbital groove and canal and emerges on the face through the infraorbital foramen. It supplies the skin of the lower eyelid, front of the cheek, and side of the nose. The zygomatic nerve enters the orbit through the inferior orbital fissure. It divides into two branches—the zygomaticotemporal and the zygomaticofacial nerves. The temporal portion pierces the zygomatic bone and distributes to the skin of the temple. The facial branch emerges on the face through a foramen in the zygomatic bone and supplies the skin on the prominence of the cheek.

The superior alveolar nerves are three in number—posterior, middle, and anterior. The posterior superior nerve arises from the maxillary nerve in the pterygopalatine fossa and descends to enter the superior alveolar foramen on the back of the maxilla. The middle and anterior superior alveolar nerves arise from the infraorbital nerve in the infraorbital groove. They communicate with the posterior nerve to form a plexus that supplies the maxillary teeth and gingiva. In general, the posterior supplies the molar teeth, the middle supplies the premolars, and the anterior supplies the canines and incisors. All three alveolar branches come to lie within the lining of the maxillary sinus and supply branches to it.

The greater palatine branch of the maxillary nerve enters the greater palatine canal, where it divides into nasal branches and the greater and lesser palatine nerves. The nasal nerves supply the nasal mucosa, while the palatine nerves enter the palate through the greater and lesser palatine foramina and supply the palate and gingiva. The lesser palatine nerves supply the soft palate, while the greater palatine nerves course anteriorly to supply the hard palate and associated gingiva. One of the nasal branches, the nasopalatine nerve, supplies the nose and then enters the palate anteriorly through the incisive canal. There it supplies the anterior palatal mucosa and gingiva (Figure 5–10). The pterygopalatine ganglion is attached to the maxillary nerve in the pterygopalatine fossa. It is an autonomic, not sensory, ganglion, and its function will be discussed presently.

The Mandibular Nerve.   The large mandibular division of the trigeminal nerve is both sensory and motor (Figure 5–11). It supplies motor innervation to the muscles of mastication, the mylohyoid, and the anterior belly of the digastric. It is sensory to the anterior two thirds of the tongue, the floor of the mouth, the buccal mucosa, the mandibular teeth, and the skin of the temporal region, lateral cheek, mandible, chin, and lower lip.

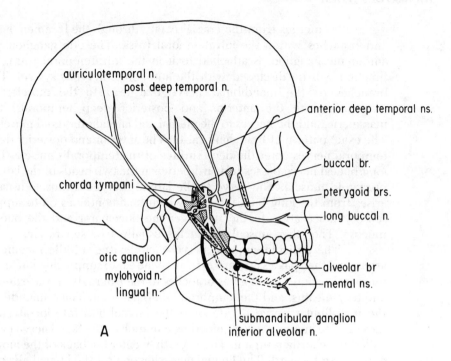

A

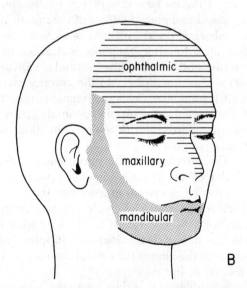

B

FIGURE 5–11   (A) mandibular division of the trigeminal nerve; (B) diagram of the sensory distribution of the trigeminal nerve on the face.

It emerges from the cranial cavity through the foramen ovale and branches within the infratemporal fossa. The otic ganglion, an autonomic ganglion, is attached to it in the infratemporal fossa. Its function will be discussed with the autonomic nervous system. The branches of the mandibular nerve that lead to the muscles of mastication are the anterior and posterior deep temporals, the masseteric, and the nerves to the medial and lateral pterygoid muscles. The exact pattern of branching varies. The anterior and posterior deep temporal nerves enter the deep surface of the temporalis muscle. The long buccal nerve passes forward between the two heads of the lateral pterygoid muscle. The nerve to the lateral pterygoid muscle usually arises from the long buccal nerve, which then continues on to supply sensory innervation to the skin over the buccinator and the buccal mucosa. The other muscular branches usually arise separately.

The auriculotemporal nerve encircles the middle meningeal artery and then passes upward in front of the ear to supply the skin of the temporal region. It also gives branches to the external ear, the external auditory meatus, and the temporomandibular joint. The remainder of the mandibular nerve divides into the lingual and inferior alveolar nerves. The lingual nerve is joined by a branch of the facial nerve (VII) called the chorda tympani. Together, they enter the back of the mouth and course forward. The lingual nerve lies against the lingual alveolar processes of the molar teeth. It then passes above the submandibular salivary gland and onto the floor of the mouth and undersurface of the tongue, where it breaks up into branches. The small submandibular ganglion, an autonomic ganglion, is attached to the lingual nerve near the anterior end of the submandibular salivary gland. The chorda tympani carries taste fibers to the anterior two thirds of the tongue. Although it hitchhikes with the lingual nerve, it is a part of the facial nerve. The lingual nerve supplies general sensory fibers (not taste) to the anterior two thirds of the tongue, the floor of the mouth, and the mandibular gingiva.

The inferior alveolar nerve enters the mandible through the mandibular canal. The mylohyoid nerve is given off just before the inferior alveolar nerve disappears into the jaw. The mylohyoid nerve runs forward in the mylohyoid groove, supplying the muscle and anterior belly of the digastric. The inferior alveolar nerve travels through the mandibular canal and supplies the mandibular teeth. It emerges onto the chin at the mental foramen and supplies the skin of the chin and lower lip.

It is obvious that damage to the trigeminal ganglion or any one of the three divisions of the nerve has serious consequences. Loss of the ophthalmic division results in loss of the corneal reflex on the affected side because the sensory innervation of the cornea is supplied by the ophthalmic nerve. Loss of the maxillary nerve would result in the loss of sensory innervation of the maxillary teeth and middle face of the affected side. Loss of function of the mandibular nerve would result in paralysis of the muscles of mastication on the affected side and loss of sensory innervation to the tongue, teeth, and lower face.

Pain in one of the branches of a division of the trigeminal is often referred to the other branches of that division. A carious mandibular tooth can result in pain in the ear. Likewise, a carious maxillary tooth may result in pain in the eye. Trigeminal neuralgia, or tic douloureaux, is a disorder that may involve one or more divisions of the trigeminal. The disease consists of extremely severe pain over the distribution of the division. The cause and cure are unknown.

The Facial Nerve (VII).   The facial nerve (VII) is both sensory and motor (Figure 5-12). The sensory portion provides taste to the anterior two thirds of the tongue as the chorda tympani. The sensory ganglion of the facial nerve is the geniculate ganglion. It is located in the petrous temporal bone near the middle ear. The unipolar cells send a central fiber through the internal auditory meatus to the brain stem at the junction of the medulla and pons. The peripheral fibers from the geniculate ganglion form the chorda tympani, exit the ear through a

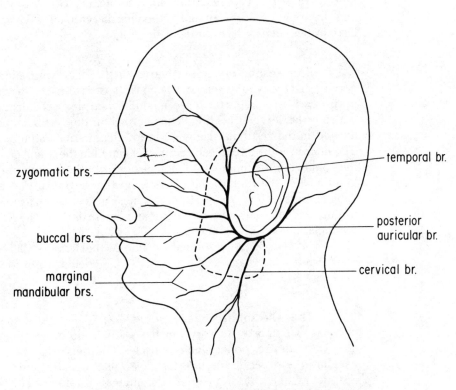

FIGURE 5-12   Motor distribution of the facial nerve.

small foramen, and join with the lingual nerve as previously described. They then travel with the lingual nerve to the tongue, supplying the tastebuds on the anterior two thirds of the tongue.

The motor root of the facial nerve arises from the brain stem and enters the ear through the internal auditory meatus. The fibers pass through the ear and out the stylomastoid foramen. Just after emerging, the nerve gives branches to the posterior belly of the digastric and the stylohyoid muscles.

The facial nerve enters the face in the substance of the parotid gland. It divides into branches that supply the muscles of facial expression. These branches are the temporal, zygomatic, buccal, marginal mandibular, and cervical. The temporal branches supply the ear muscles, the frontalis, and the lateral eye muscles. The zygomatic branches supply the orbicularis oculi. The buccal branches innervate the muscles in the middle of the face. The marginal mandibular nerves innervate the muscles of the lower face and the cervical branch supplies the platysma.

Surgery or pathology of the parotid may result in damage to the facial nerve or some of its branches. Damage to the motor portion of the facial nerve results in Bell's Palsy on the affected side. The muscles of facial expression become paralyzed, resulting in an expressionless face and drooping mouth. Damage to the chorda tympani results in loss of taste in the anterior two thirds of the tongue.

The Vestibulocochlear Nerve (VIII).   The vestibulocochlear nerve (VIII) is wholly sensory. It consists of two parts—a vestibular portion, which conveys the sense of equilibrium, and a cochlear portion, which is the nerve of hearing. The neurons for the vestibular nerve are located in the vestibular ganglion inside the internal auditory meatus. The neurons of the cochlear nerve are located in the spinal ganglion of the cochlea in the inner ear. The neurons of both portions are bipolar like those of the retina. The fibers from the vestibular and cochlear ganglia unite to form the vestibulocochlear nerve, which leaves the ear through the internal auditory meatus and enters the brain stem lateral to the facial nerve.

Section of the vestibular portion of the nerve results in loss of equilibrium and nausea. Damage to the cochlear portion causes deafness.

The Glossopharyngeal Nerve (IX).   The glossopharyngeal nerve (IX) is mostly sensory but has a small motor component that innervates the stylopharyngeus muscle. The nerve has two sensory ganglia—the superior and inferior glossopharyngeal ganglia. They lie just below the exterior rim of the jugular foramen. The superior ganglion may be within the jugular foramen. The central fibers from the ganglia enter the cranial cavity through the jugular foramen and enter the medulla just behind the vestibulocochlear nerve. The motor fibers follow the reverse route, join with the peripheral sensory fibers, and pass between the internal carotid and internal jugular to enter the pharynx. Here, the nerve supplies taste fibers to the posterior one third of the tongue and general sensory innervation to the epiglottis, the root of the tongue, the soft palate, and the pharynx. Branches of the glossopharyngeal join with contributions from the vagus (X) and spinal accessory (XI) nerves to form the pharyngeal plexus.

Section of the glossopharyngeal results in loss of taste to the posterior one third of the tongue and loss of the gag reflex, which requires feeling in the throat to function.

The Vagus Nerve (X).   The vagus nerve has the longest course and distribution of all the cranial nerves. It is both sensory and motor. The sensory ganglia are the superior (jugular) and inferior (nodose). Like the glossopharyngeal, they are located near the inferior opening of the jugular foramen. The cells of the ganglia send a central process through the jugular foramen into the medulla behind the ninth cranial nerve. The motor component arises here and, passing through the jugular foramen and ganglia, joins the peripheral fibers from the sensory neurons to form the peripheral nerve. The vagus then descends between the internal carotid artery and the internal jugular vein into and through the chest to the abdominal cavity. It has many branches in the chest and abdomen, but we will only consider the branches in the neck.

A small auricular branch supplies sensory innervation to the external ear. The vagus is joined by part of the spinal accessory nerve (XI). It is these fibers disguised as the vagus nerve that supply motor innervation to the muscles of the soft palate (except the tensor palatini) and pharynx through branches to the pharyngeal plexus. The superior laryngeal and recurrent laryngeal nerves of the vagus supply the larynx. The superior nerve is sensory to the mucosa of the larynx above the vocal cords. It also contains some taste fibers to tastebuds on the epiglottis.

The recurrent laryngeal supplies vagal motor fibers to the laryngeal muscles and also sensory fibers to the laryngeal mucosa below the vocal cords. The recurrent nerves are so named because, during development, they become hooked around the subclavian artery on the right and the arch of the aorta on the left and are pulled down toward the chest, from which position they must "recur" upward to enter the larynx. Great care must be taken to avoid sectioning or damaging the nerves during surgery on the larynx or thyroid gland. Damage would result in loss of speech or difficulty in speaking. Loss of the sensory component of the vagus has little effect in the head but results in the loss of visceral sensation and of many reflexes such as the cough, gag, and vomit reflexes.

The Spinal Accessory Nerve (XI).   The spinal accessory (XI) nerve is motor and has two roots, one from the spinal cord (spinal root) and one from the medulla (cranial root) posterior to the tenth cranial nerve. The spinal rootlets join to form a trunk that enters the skull through the foramen magnum. The trunk is joined by fibers of the cranial root from the medulla. The two portions unite just long enough to exit through the jugular foramen. The cranial root then joins the vagus nerve and contributes to the pharyngeal plexus. The spinal portion gives motor innervation to the trapezius and sternocleidomastoid muscles. Damage to this nerve results in difficulty in rotating the head.

The Hypoglossal Nerve (XII).   The hypoglossal nerve (XII) is entirely motor in function. It innervates the intrinsic and extrinsic muscles of the tongue except the palatoglossus muscle. It arises from the medulla and exits the cranial cavity in the hypoglossal canal. It curves forward and enters the posterior of the mouth above the hyoid bone. Section or damage results in paralysis of the tongue. When the tongue is protruded, it deviates toward the damaged side.

TABLE 5–1. Summary of Cranial Nerves

Cranial Nerve and Number	Sensory (S) Motor (M)	Sensory Ganglion	Areas Supplied, Function	Pathology
Olfactory (I)	S	Olfactory epith.	Sense of smell	Anosmia
Optic (II)	S	Retina	Sight	Blindness, optic defects
Oculomotor (III)	M	—	Extrinsic muscles of the eye (Superior, inferior, and medial rectus muscles and inferior oblique)	Deviation of the eyeball
Trochlear (IV)	M	—	Superior oblique muscle of the eye	Deviation of the eyeball
Trigeminal (V)	S	Semilunar	Skin of face and scalp, mucosa of the nose and mouth, teeth	Loss of general sense in these structures
	M	—	Muscles of mastication, tensor veli palatini, mylohyoid, ant. belly of digastric	Paralysis of these muscles
Abducens (VI)	M	—	Lateral rectus muscle of the eye	Deviation of the eyeball

TABLE 5–1. Summary of Cranial Nerves (continued)

Cranial Nerve and Number	Sensory (S) Motor (M)	Sensory Ganglion	Areas Supplied, Function	Pathology
Facial (VII)	S	Geniculate	Skin in the region of the ear, chorda tympani	Loss of general sense in this region, loss of taste, anterior 2/3rds of tongue
	M	—	Muscles of facial expression stylo-hyoid and post. belly of digastric	Bell's palsy
Vestibulo-cochlear (VIII)	S	Cochlea Vestibular apparatus	Sense of hearing Sense of balance	Deafness Vertigo, dizziness
Glossopharyngeal (IX)	S	Superior and inferior	General sense on the post. 1/3 of the tongue, epiglottis, soft palate, pharynx; taste on post. 1/3 of tongue	Loss of taste and general sense on post. 1/3 of tongue, loss of general sense on soft palate and pharynx
	M	—	Stylopharyngeus muscle	Paralysis of stylo-pharyngeus
Vagus (X)	S	Superior (jugular) inferior (nodose)	Pharynx through pharyngeal plexus, mucosa of larynx	Possible loss of some reflexes
	M	—	Muscles of larynx	Loss of speech, difficulty speaking
Spinal accessory (XI)	M	—	Trapezius, sterno-cleidomastoid, pharynx through pharyngeal plexus	Difficulty rotating head
Hypoglossal (XII)	M	—	Intrinsic and ex-trinsic muscles of the tongue except the palatoglossus	Paralysis of the tongue

THE AUTONOMIC NERVOUS SYSTEM

The autonomic nervous system is often referred to as the "automatic" nervous system because it regulates many body functions such as heart rate, respiratory rate, diameter of blood vessels, glandular secretion, and visceral functions, without conscious effort. The system is purely motor and consists of two divisions: the sympathetic and parasympathetic systems.

While the two divisions often have opposing functions, they have some anatomic characteristics in common. The autonomic nervous system is a two-neuron system. The first neuron is located in the brain or spinal cord. The second neuron is located in a ganglion outside the brain or spinal cord. The first neuron sends out a fiber, called the preganglionic fiber, which makes contact (synapses) with the second neuron in a ganglion. The second neuron, in the ganglion, then sends out a postganglionic fiber, which innervates the target organ. The anatomic difference between the sympathetic and parasympathetic divisions is simply the location of the first and second neurons.

The Sympathetic Nervous System

The sympathetic nervous system is often called the thoracolumbar system because the first neuron is located in the spinal cord in the thoracic and lumbar regions (Figure 5–13). The second neuron is located in one of the sympathetic chain ganglia. These ganglia are located on either side of the spinal column on the posterior body wall in the thorax, abdomen, and pelvis and on either side of the anterior surface of the cervical vertebral column. The ganglia are attached to each other, forming a paired chain on either side of the spinal column.

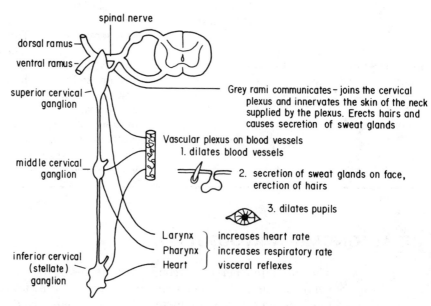

FIGURE 5–13   The sympathetic nervous system in the head.

The preganglionic fibers leave the spinal cord with the ventral root of each thoracic and first lumbar spinal nerve. They then separate from the nerve and enter the sympathetic chain. These preganglionic fibers going from the spinal nerves to the sympathetic chain are called the white rami communicantes because the fibers are myelinated. Some fibers synapse immediately, while others go up or down the chain before synapsing.

The sympathetic chain has three ganglia in the neck and several in the pelvis. These ganglia are simply extensions of the chain. The preganglionic fibers that reach these ganglia originate in the thoracic and lumbar spinal cord and travel up or down the chain to reach the cervical and pelvic ganglia. Following synapse, the second neuron, located in the sympathetic chain, sends out a fiber to the target organ. These fibers are usually not myelinated and rejoin the spinal nerve to be distributed with it. The short bundles of postganglionic fibers connecting the chain to spinal nerves are called the gray rami communicantes. In the sympathetic system, the preganglionic (first) fiber is usually short, and the postganglionic (second) fiber is usually long.

The Parasympathetic Nervous System

The parasympathetic nervous system is sometimes called the craniosacral system. The first neuron is located in the medulla of the brain or the sacral spinal cord. Fibers from the first neuron (preganglionic) exit the brain with a cranial nerve or exit the sacral spinal cord with the ventral root of the sacral spinal nerves. The second neuron is located in a ganglion very near the organ to be innervated, so the preganglionic fiber of the parasympathetic system is usually long, and the postganglionic fiber is quite short.

Autonomics of the Head and Neck

Sympathetic Nervous System. The sympathetic chain in the head and neck consists of three ganglia: the superior cervical ganglion, the middle cervical ganglion, and the inferior or stellate ganglion. The middle cervical ganglion is often absent. Preganglionic fibers from the thoracic spinal cord synapse with cells in the cervical sympathetic ganglia. Postganglionic fibers from the cells in the ganglia take one of three courses. Some postganglionic fibers from each ganglion form plexes along neighboring blood vessels like the carotid, vertebral, and subclavian arteries. In this manner, they innervate the blood vessels of the head and neck and hitchhike to destinations such as the orbit, which is reached via the internal carotid artery.

In addition, some postganglionic fibers from each cervical sympathetic ganglion form gray rami communicantes, which join the cervical spinal nerves and distribute with them via the cervical plexus to the skin of the neck. Finally, some postganglionic fibers leave the ganglia and travel, unaided, to the viscera. In this manner, postganglionic sympathetic fibers reach the pharyngeal plexus, esophagus, trachea, thyroid gland, parathyroid glands, and heart. Stimulation of the sympathetic nervous system dilates the pupils, causes sweating, dilates blood vessels, increases respiration and heart rate, and decreases gastric activity and salivation.

Parasympathetic Nervous System. The preganglionic neurons of the parasympathetic nervous system in the head arise near, and are associated with, three cranial nerves: the oculomotor, the glossopharyngeal, and the facial (Table 5–2). The postganglionic neurons are located in named parasympathetic ganglia near the target organ. The parasympathetic fibers hitchhike on the cranial nerves to get where they must go. Do not confuse the parasympathetic ganglia of the head with the sensory ganglia of the cranial nerves. The autonomic ganglia are located along the course of the cranial nerves, but the fibers of the cranial nerves simply pass through.

Preganglionic parasympathetic fibers associated with the oculomotor nerve arise near its origin in the medulla. They pass into the orbit with the nerve and synapse in the tiny ciliary ganglion in the orbit. The postganglionic fibers from the ciliary ganglion innervate the ciliary muscle and sphincter muscle of the pupil. These fibers are responsible for accommodation of the lens and constriction of the pupil.

The preganglionic fibers associated with the glossopharyngeal nerve arise near its origin in the medulla. They enter the ear and become known as the lesser petrosal nerve. When they exit the ear near the chorda tympani, they synapse in the otic ganglion. Postganglionic fibers from the otic ganglion then go to the parotid salivary gland in the auriculotemporal branch of the trigeminal nerve. Stimulation of these nerves causes a copious flow of watery saliva from that gland.

Preganglionic fibers arising in company with the facial nerve take one of two courses. Some accompany the chorda tympani to the submandibular ganglion. Postganglionic fibers from the submandibular ganglion supply the submandibular and sublingual salivary glands and glands of the tongue. Again, stimulation produces copious salivation. A second group of preganglionic fibers becomes the greater petrosal nerve and passes to the pterygopalatine ganglion. The postganglionic fibers from the pterygopalatine pass to the glands of the pharynx, palate, and also to the lacrimal gland in branches of the trigeminal nerve. Stimulation results in secretion of these glands.

Visceral Sensory Nerves. In order for the autonomic nerves to carry out their functions, they must be connected to sensory neurons, which tell them when there is a need to act. The sensory fibers involved belong to the neurons of the dorsal root ganglia or sensory ganglia of the cranial nerves. The means by which the sensory information is relayed to the autonomic motor neurons involves complex systems within the brain and spinal cord.

TABLE 5–2. Pathways of Parasympathetic Nerves

Name of Origin	Preganglionic Nerve	Ganglion	Postganglionic Nerve	Organ Innervated, Function
Oculomotor nerve	—	Ciliary	—	Pupillary muscle, constricts pupil Ciliary muscle, stretches and thins the lens of the eye
Facial nerve (motor root)	A. Chorda tympani	Submandibular	—	Submandibular and sublingual salivary glands and glands of the tongue, stimulates secretion
	B. Greater petrosal	Pterygopalatine	$V_{MAX.}$	Pharyngeal and palatine salivary glands and lacrimal glands, stimulates secretion
Glossopharyngeal nerve	Lesser petrosal n.	Otic	Ariculotemporal br. of $V_{MAND.}$	Parotid gland, stimulates secretion

STUDY EXERCISES

1. Diagram a cross-section of the cervical spinal cord and spinal nerve.
2. Where are the cell bodies of sensory neurons located? Where are the cell bodies of motor neurons located?
3. *Briefly describe the distribution of the dorsal rami of the cervical spinal nerves.*
4. What happens to the ventral rami of the cervical spinal nerves?
5. List the names and numbers of the cranial nerves in order.
6. Give the name and number of the cranial nerve associated with each of the following:

    A. Motor to the intrinsic muscles of the tongue
    B. Motor to the muscles of facial expression
    C. Semilunar ganglion
    D. Cochlea
    E. Motor to the superior oblique muscle of the eye
    F. Sense of balance
    G. Geniculate ganglion
    H. Motor to the muscles of the larynx
    I. Motor to the muscles of mastication
    J. Motor to the sternocleidomastoid muscle

7. How are the sympathetic and parasympathetic nervous systems similar? How are they different?
8. What does the sympathetic nervous system do in the head and neck?
9. What three cranial nerves are associated with the parasympathetic nervous system in the head and neck?
10. Name the four parasympathetic ganglia of the head and neck.
11. What are the functions of the parasympathetic nervous system in the head and neck?

6

THE
RESPIRATORY
SYSTEM

LEARNING OBJECTIVES

At the conclusion of this chapter, the student should be able to:

1. Describe the anatomic features of the oral cavity.
2. Describe the tongue including its surface features and intrinsic musculature.
3. Understand the structures within the nasal cavities.
4. Learn the names and locations of the paranasal sinuses.
5. Know the functional relationship of the maxillary sinus to the maxillary molar teeth.
6. Learn the names and locations of the cartilages of the larynx.
7. Know the location and attachments of the vocal cords and the significance of laryngospasm.

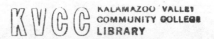

The respiratory system of the head and neck consists of the oral cavity, nasal cavities, paranasal sinuses, larynx, and trachea.

THE ORAL CAVITY

The oral cavity may be divided into the vestibule and oral cavity proper. The vestibule is the space between the teeth and cheeks, laterally, and the lips anteriorly. The oral cavity proper is the space bounded by the alveolar arches, the floor of the mouth, and the palate. It ends posteriorly at the entrance to the oral pharynx. The vestibule communicates with the oral cavity behind the last molar teeth and extraorally through the lips (labia).

The line of contact of the closed lips is the oral fissure. A depression in the center of the external surface of the upper lip, the philtrum, ends in a small protrusion, the tubercle. The pink portion of the lips between the skin on the outside and the oral mucosa is called the vermilion zone. The lips are composed of the orbicularis oris muscle and connective tissue. They are continuous with the cheeks, and the junction is marked externally by the nasolabial sulcus running from the side of the nose to the angle of the mouth. Each lip is connected to the alveolar mucosa by a small fold of mucous membrane, the labial frenulum.

The cheeks are composed of the buccinator muscle, some muscles of facial expression, and a variable amount of fat and connective tissue. The lining mucosa contains a number of small buccal salivary glands. The duct of the parotid gland enters the mouth, piercing the buccinator next to the maxillary second molar, and ends on a small papilla.

Much of the oral cavity proper is occupied by the tongue (Figure 6–1). The posterior attachment is called the root of the tongue, and the tip is called the apex. The upper surface is the dorsum. The tongue is a muscle and is composed of muscle fibers that run longitudinally, transversely, and vertically. The longitudinal fibers may be divided into superior and inferior groups that extend from root to apex under the mucosa of the dorsum and undersurface respectively. A connective tissue septum in the median longitudinal plane gives origin to the transverse fibers, which pass laterally to the borders of the tongue. Vertical fibers are located at the sides of the middle to apical region of the tongue. They run from the dorsum to the underside. The intrinsic and extrinsic muscles of the tongue give it the very great range of movement necessary for its complex role in chewing, swallowing, and speech.

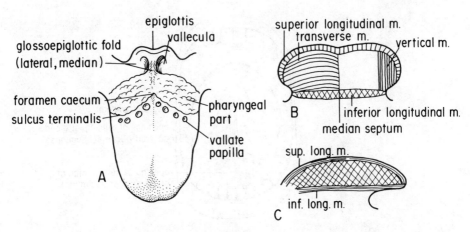

FIGURE 6-1 (A) dorsal surface of the tongue; (B) diagram of a transverse section through the tongue showing intrinsic musculature; (C) diagram of a longitudinal section of the tongue.

The posterior one third of the tongue is separated from the anterior two thirds by a "V"-shaped sulcus, the sulcus terminalis. The mucosa of the tongue anterior to the sulcus contains many papillae, which give the tongue its soft feel. Some of the papillae contain tastebuds. A row of very large vallate papillae are located just anterior to the sulcus. The vallate papillae are so named because each is surrounded by a small valley or crypt. A small pit, the foramen caecum, may be found at the point of the "V" of the sulcus terminalis. This is the site of origin of the thyroid gland during development. Some tonsilar tissue, the lingual tonsil, may be found at the posterior part of the tongue also. A single median and two lateral glossoepiglottic folds extend from the root of the tongue to the epiglottis. The small depression between the median fold and each lateral fold is called the vallecula.

The tongue is connected to the floor of the mouth anteriorly by the lingual frenulum (Figure 6-2). At the base of the frenulum are two small papillae, the salivary caruncles. They are the site of entry of the duct of the submandibular salivary gland. A ridge in the sublingual mucosa extends posteriorly from the caruncles. This is the sublingual fold (plicae sublingualis). The sublingual salivary glands lie beneath and open along this fold.

The palate forms the roof of the oral cavity (Figure 6-3). The hard palate presents a median ridge, the raphe, and numerous small ridges perpendicular to it, the rugae. The raphe is the line of fusion of the maxillary processes of the palate. A small papilla, the nasopalatine

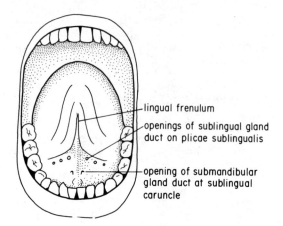

FIGURE 6–2   Sublingual area of the oral cavity.

lingual frenulum

openings of sublingual gland duct on plicae sublingualis

opening of submandibular gland duct at sublingual caruncle

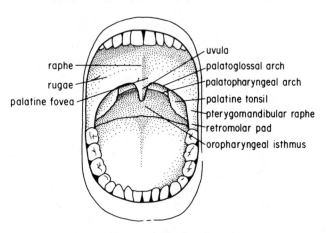

FIGURE 6–3   The oral cavity.

raphe

rugae

palatine fovea

uvula

palatoglossal arch

palatopharyngeal arch

palatine tonsil

pterygomandibular raphe

retromolar pad

oropharyngeal isthmus

(incisive) papilla, marks the site of the nasopalatine or incisive foramen at the anterior end of the raphe. Posteriorly, at the junction of the hard and soft palates near the midline, are two small pits, the palatine fovea. A small fleshy protuberance, the uvula, hangs from the midline of the soft palate. Two pairs of folds of mucosa arch from the palate to the tongue on either side of the opening into the oral pharynx. The more anterior folds form the palatoglossal arch and contain the palatoglossus muscle. This arch marks the oropharyngeal isthmus or fauces. The palatopharyngeal arch curves behind the palatoglossal arch and contains the palatopharyngeus muscle. The space between the arches on either side is occupied by the palatine tonsil.

A third and less prominent fold begins behind the last mandibular molar tooth in a fleshy pad called the retromolar pad. It arches upward to the palate. The pterygomandibular raphe is beneath the mucosa at this location.

THE NASAL CAVITIES

The paired nasal cavities are separated from one another by the nasal septum. The septum is partly bony and partly cartilaginous and forms the medial wall of each cavity (Figure 6–4). The bony portion is formed by the vomer and perpendicular plate of the ethmoid as previously described. The gap between these bones anteriorly is filled by the septal cartilage. The nose communicates with the external environment through the nostrils. The posterior openings into the nasopharynx are the choanae. The roof of each nasal cavity is bounded by the ethmoid bone and houses the olfactory epithelium.

The lateral walls of the cavities have three bony projections: the superior, middle, and inferior nasal conchae. They are curved, scroll-like processes. The superior and middle conchae are processes of the ethmoid bone. The inferior concha is a separate bone that articulates with the lateral nasal wall. The narrow, slit-like space beneath each concha is called a meatus. The paranasal sinuses drain into the nasal cavities within the meatuses. The posterior ethmoid air cells open into the superior meatus. The middle meatus contains a sickle-shaped slit,

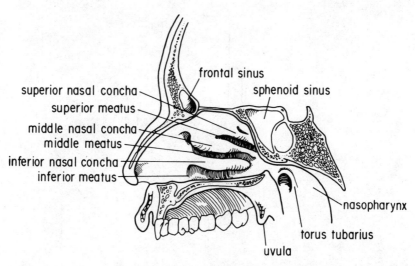

FIGURE 6–4   Sagittal section of the head showing the nasal wall.

the hiatus semilunaris. The frontal and maxillary sinuses and anterior ethmoid air cells open into the hiatus and thus the middle meatus. In addition, the middle ethmoid air cells open independently into the middle meatus. The nasolacrimal duct, which drains tears from the eyes, opens into the inferior meatus.

The opening of the auditory tube (Eustachian tube) lies just behind the posterior end of the inferior nasal conchae. The opening is hooded by a bump, the torus tubarius, formed by the tubal cartilage. The pharyngeal tonsil is located in the pharyngeal wall opposite the auditory opening.

THE PARANASAL SINUSES

The paranasal sinuses are spaces in the frontal, ethmoid, sphenoid, and maxillary bones (Figure 6-5). They develop as evaginations of the lateral nasal wall and are lined with mucosa that is continuous with that of the nasal cavities. They continue to enlarge slowly throughout life and can become quite extensive.

The frontal sinuses are located in the frontal bone on either side of the midline above the superciliary arch. They are roughly triangular and are seldom symmetrical. They open into the middle nasal meatus.

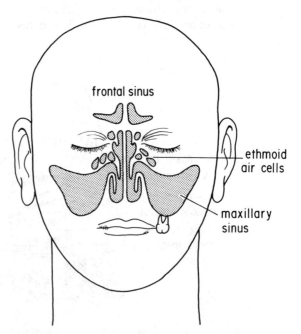

FIGURE 6–5   Diagram of the paranasal sinuses.

The ethmoid air cells are thin-walled, honeycombed chambers in the ethmoid bone. Their numbers vary, and they are usually divided into anterior, middle, and posterior groups that communicate with the nasal meatuses as previously described.

The sphenoid sinuses are cuboidal spaces on either side of the midline in the body of the sphenoid bone. They open into the nasal cavities above and behind the superior nasal conchae.

The maxillary sinuses are the largest of the paranasal sinuses. They are roughly pyramidal; the point of the pyramid is directed toward the zygomatic process of the maxillary bone, and the base is roughly parallel to the lateral nasal wall. The floor of each sinus is thin and overlies the roots of the maxillary molars. Occasionally, the root of a tooth will perforate the sinus, or the sinus may be inadvertently perforated during dental procedures. Periapical abscesses involving maxillary molar teeth can penetrate and involve the maxillary sinus. Conversely, infections of the maxillary sinuses often result in pain in the molar teeth.

The communication of the maxillary sinuses with the nasal cavity is through an opening that is considerably higher than the floor of the sinus. The sinus does not drain well in the erect position. The head must be laid on one side.

THE LARYNX

The larynx is the organ of phonation. It allows air to pass into the trachea and the lungs. It is continuous above with the laryngopharynx and below with the trachea. It is covered anteriorly by the thyroid gland and infrahyoid muscles. The esophagus passes behind the larynx.

The larynx is composed of cartilages and muscles (Figures 6-6, 6-7, 6-8, and 6-9). The cartilages are the epiglottic, thyroid, cricoid, arytenoid, corniculate, and cuneiform. The epiglottic cartilage forms the substance of the epiglottis. It is flat and ovoid, or leaf-like, and attaches to the inner surface of the thyroid cartilage. The thyroid cartilage is shield-shaped and is the largest of the laryngeal cartilages. The two sides, or alae, are joined in front forming the laryngeal prominence, or Adam's apple. The sides curve backward and upward. Superior and inferior horns or cornua project upward and downward from its posterior margin.

The cricoid cartilage is shaped like a signet ring, wide posteriorly and narrow anteriorly. The thyroid and cricoid cartilages articulate in joints between the inferior cornu of the thyroid and a small articular facet on each side of the cricoid.

The paired arytenoid cartilages are small and roughly pyramidal. They sit on top of the posterior superior border of the cricoid.

The vocal cords attach to a process of the arytenoid called the vocal process.

The corniculate cartilages are two small nodules that sit on the tips of the arytenoids. The cuneiform cartilages are small, slender, and curved. They occupy the posterior edge of the opening of the larynx and do not articulate with the other cartilages.

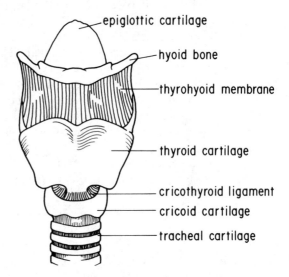

FIGURE 6–6   Anterior aspect of the larynx.

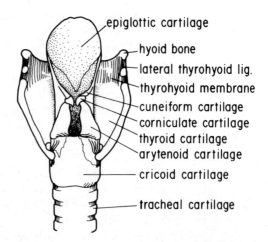

FIGURE 6–7   Posterior aspect of the laryngeal cartilages.

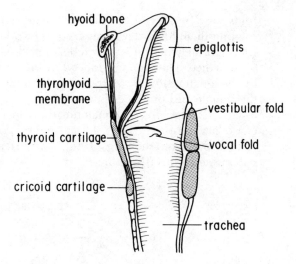

hyoid bone

epiglottis

thyrohyoid membrane

vestibular fold

thyroid cartilage

vocal fold

cricoid cartilage

trachea

FIGURE 6–8   Sagittal section of the larynx.

The space on the front of the larynx between the thyroid and cricoid cartilages is closed by connective tissue called the cricothyroid membrane. The space between the upper anterior edge of the thyroid cartilage and the lower anterior edge of the hyoid bone is occupied by the thyrohyoid membrane. The thickening in this membrane between the superior cornua of the thyroid cartilage and the tip of its greater horn of the hyoid bone is called the lateral thyrohyoid ligament.

Most of the cartilages of the larynx are covered by muscles and mucosa that give the larynx a smooth, conical appearance from behind. If the interior of the larynx is viewed from above, as with a laryngoscope, two sets of folds are visible projecting from the sides of the larynx (Figures 6–8 and 6–9). The upper pair are called the vestibular folds and the opening between them, the rimi vestibuli. The lower folds are the vocal folds, commonly called the vocal cords. The opening between them is the rima glottidis. The medial edge of the vestibular fold is thickened and contains the vestibular ligament. It is attached to the depression between the two alae of the thyroid cartilage in front and to the arytenoid cartilage behind. The vocal folds contain the vocalis muscle. Their medial edges project further into the laryngeal cavity than the vestibular folds. The medial edge of the vocal fold contains the vocal ligament. The vocal ligament is attached to the center of the thyroid cartilage anteriorly and the vocal process of the arytenoid cartilage posteriorly.

Tension on the vocal folds and the distance between them can be varied. The cricoid cartilage can rotate up and down at the cricothyroid joint, tensing or relaxing the vocal folds. The distance between the folds may be altered by moving the arytenoid cartilages apart or by rotating them toward or away from each other (Figure 6–9). The vocal folds vibrate when air is passed between them. This produces the sound of the voice. The sound produced by the vibrating folds is then shaped by the tongue and lips to produce speech. The male larynx is larger than the female and produces lower tones.

Foreign objects contacting the upper larynx or vocal folds may cause laryngospasm. The folds are tightly apposed to prevent passage of the object into the lungs. If the spasm is allowed to continue, death will ensue from suffocation.

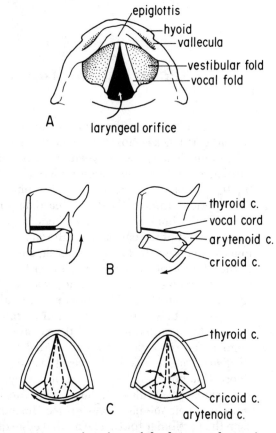

FIGURE 6–9 (A) superior view of the laryngeal opening; (B) diagram of the movement of the cricoid cartilage and its effect on the vocal cords; (C) diagram of the movements of the arytenoid cartilages and their effect on the size of the laryngeal opening.

STUDY EXERCISES

1. Using a mirror, find the following structures described for the oral cavity:

   A. Palatoglossal arch
   B. Palatopharyngeal arch
   C. Pterygomandibular raphe
   D. Retromolar pad
   E. Labial and lingual frenula
   F. Openings of the major salivary glands

2. Move your tongue over your hard palate. Can you feel the rugae? Can you feel the palatal raphe?

3. Observe the dorsum of the tongue. Note the distribution of the different types of papillae. Find the sulcus terminalis, foramen caecum, and lingual tonsil.

4. Tap lightly over the area of the frontal sinuses and then on the forehead above the sinuses. Note the difference in sound. The sinuses should produce a lower, slightly hollow sound. Tap on the maxillary sinus. The maxillary sinus may be transilluminated by placing a small flashlight near the bottom of the sinus in a darkened room. The cavity of the sinus will be dully lit. If the sinus is partially filled with mucus or pus, as in a cold or infection, less light will be transmitted. Try transilluminating prepared skulls present in your classroom.

5. Name the major cartilages of the larynx. *How are the vocal cords attached, and how do the movements of the cartilages change the sound produced?*

6. What happens if something touches the vocal or vestibular folds?

7

GLANDS OF
THE HEAD
AND NECK

LEARNING OBJECTIVES

At the conclusion of this chapter, the student should be able to:

1. Describe the location of the three major salivary glands, and give the name of each duct, its course, and its opening.
2. Appreciate the location and function of the thyroid, parathyroid, pituitary, and lacrimal glands.

SALIVARY GLANDS

There are three major salivary glands and a number of minor glands as well (Figure 7-1). The parotid gland is the largest salivary gland. It covers the angle of the jaw and extends behind the earlobe. It ends superiorly at the lower edge of the zygomatic arch in front of the ear. It extends onto the masseter as far as the middle of the muscle. The duct, Stensen's duct, exits the middle of the anterior edge of the gland. It crosses the masseter and pierces the buccinator to enter the mouth opposite the second maxillary molar tooth. A small amount of glandular tissue located on the duct is called the accessory parotid.

The gland is encapsulated, and several structures run in it. The retromandibular vein, the superficial temporal artery, and the facial nerve all pierce the substance of the gland and branch with it.

The submandibular salivary gland has a deep and a superficial part. The smaller, deep portion is deep to the mylohyoid muscle. The superficial portion lies on the mylohyoid between the digastric muscle and the mandible. The two parts are connected behind the posterior margin of the mylohyoid muscle. The submandibular gland is about the size of a walnut. Its duct, Wharton's duct, passes between the mylohyoid and hyoglossus muscles and enters the mouth at the sublingual caruncle.

The sublingual gland is not encapsulated. It lies under the sublingual mucosa beneath the sublingual fold (plica sublingualis) onto which its multiple ducts (ducts of Rivinus) empty. It may have eight to twenty ducts, some of which usually open into the submandibular duct instead of the plica.

Many minor salivary glands empty directly onto the oral mucosa. These glands are composed of a single or several secretory units. They are named the labial, buccal, palatine, and lingual, according to their location in the oral mucosa. The labial and buccal glands are relatively sparse. The palatine glands are few anteriorly but quite numerous posteriorly. The lingual glands are found in two groups. The anterior groups, glands of Blandin and Nuhn, are on the underside of the apex of the tongue, under the mucosa and inferior longitudinal muscle. They open onto the undersurface of the tongue by several small ducts. The posterior group, von Ebner's glands, are found in association with the circumvallate papillae. They open into the bottom of the crypts of the papillae and are thought to have a cleansing function.

The different glands secrete saliva of slightly different composition. The glands are composed of two types of secretory cells that produce two types of secretion. Serous cells produce a thin, watery substance, while the mucous cells produce a thick, viscous material. Together, the secretions constitute saliva. In addition, the rate of

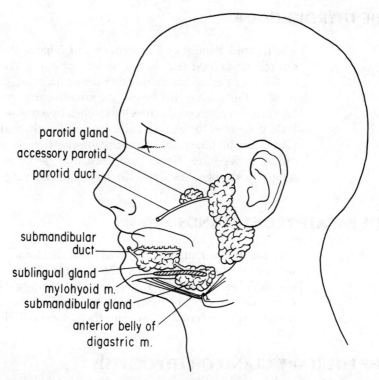

parotid gland

accessory parotid

parotid duct

submandibular duct

sublingual gland

mylohyoid m.

submandibular gland

anterior belly of digastric m.

FIGURE 7–1 Locations and ducts of the major salivary glands.

salivation and composition of the saliva are altered by nervous and hormonal influences. Stimulation of the parasympathetic nervous system results in a copious flow of saliva high in mucus and enzymes. Sympathetic stimulation produces a small amount of watery secretion with little or no organic content.

Salivary stones, sialoliths, occasionally block a duct and must be removed. These stones are small concretions that cause pain sometimes accompanied by infection. Such a blockage in a sublingual gland duct is called a ranula. Secretions build up behind the blocked duct, producing a saliva-filled sac. A similar state in one of the minor glands is called a mucocele.

Sialorrhea is an overproduction of saliva. Such a condition may occur when a patient is given parasympathetic stimulating drugs. Xerostomia, or dry mouth, is the opposite of sialorrhea. It occurs in the elderly, in people on sympathetic or anti-parasympathetic drugs, following removal of a major gland, during radiation therapy, and sometimes spontaneously. It can result in rampant caries and oral fetidis because the normal cleansing action of the saliva is absent.

THE THYROID GLAND

The thyroid gland is an endocrine gland. That is, it secretes its product directly into blood vessels, not by way of ducts. The thyroid regulates metabolic rate and has many other functions as well. It is located on the front of the trachea just below the cricoid cartilage. It consists of two lateral lobes connected across the trachea by a region called the isthmus. Enlargement of the gland is called goiter. The thyroid is highly vascular. Care must be taken not to cut the inferior thyroid vein during tracheotomy procedures. Great care must also be taken not to injure the recurrent laryngeal nerve to the larynx during surgery on the thyroid.

THE PARATHYROID GLANDS

The parathyroid glands are small nodules located on the posterior surface of the thyroid under the capsule. They are also endocrine glands. There are usually four parathyroid glands. They are concerned with calcium and phosphorus metabolism. If they are removed, the muscles will undergo tetany, and the person will die.

THE PITUITARY GLAND OR HYPOPHYSIS

The pituitary gland is the master endocrine gland. It and the hypothalamus regulate all of the endocrine glands of the body. It is attached to the hypothalamus by a slender stalk and is housed in the sella turcica of the cranial cavity. Its many functions are far too complex to consider here.

THE LACRIMAL GLAND

The lacrimal gland produces fluid to lubricate the eyeball. The lacrimal gland lies in a depression in the frontal bone just inside the upper lateral orbital rim. The ducts open into the orbit all along the junction of the upper lid and conjunctiva. The fluid drains via the lacrimal puncta, small holes in the edge of the eyelid at the medial corner of the eye. The puncta drain into the lacrimal sac, which, in turn, drains through the nasolacrimal duct into the nose.

CHAPTER SUMMARY

Glands of the Head and Neck

Gland	Location	Duct and Location of Opening	Function
Salivary			
1. Parotid	Angle of the jaw in front of and partially behind the ear	Stensen's duct, oral cavity opposite second maxillary molar tooth	Produces saliva
2. Submandibular	Wraps around the free end of the mylohyoid muscle	Wharton's duct, sublingual caruncle	Produces saliva
3. Sublingual	Under the sublingual mucosa	Ducts of Rivinus, sublingual fold and submandibular duct	Produces saliva
4. Minor salivary glands	Labial, palatine, buccal, and lingual mucosa	Directly onto labial, palatine, and buccal mucosa: undersurface of tongue (glands of Blandin and Nuhn), crypts of circumvallate papillae (von Ebner's glands)	Produces saliva
Thyroid gland	Front of the trachea below the cricoid cartilage		Regulates metabolic rate
Parathyroid glands	Under capsule on posterior surface of thyroid gland		Calcium and phosphorus metabolism
Pituitary gland (Hypophysis)	Sella turcica		Regulates other endocrine glands
Lacrimal gland	Upper lateral orbital rim	Ducts open along the junction of the upper lid and conjunctiva	Produces tears that lubricate and cleanse the eye

STUDY EXERCISES

1. Describe each major salivary gland including its location, duct, and opening in the oral cavity.
2. Try to palpate your submandibular salivary gland. The portion that can be felt in the submandibular fossa is rounded and firmly encapsulated. The extent of the parotid gland is much harder to delimit by palpation. See if you can find the extent of your own parotid gland.
3. The thyroid gland is not usually visible or easily palpable. However, an enlarged thyroid is not an uncommon occurrence. Observe your classmates and colleagues. An enlarged thyroid gland will appear as a "U"-shaped swelling just below the cricoid cartilage.
4. The parathyroid glands are embedded under the capsule of the thyroid gland. What would happen if the thyroid gland were removed? (This is how we discovered the presence of the parathyroid glands.)
5. Where is the pituitary gland located, and why is it important?
6. Describe the location of the lacrimal glands and their ducts. Why does your nose run when your eyes tear?

8

FASCIA AND
FASCIAL SPACES

LEARNING OBJECTIVES

At the conclusion of this chapter, the student should be able to:

1. Give the location and function of the superficial and deep fascias of the head and neck.
2. Describe the location and communications of the fascial spaces of the head and neck and their significance to the spread of infection.

Fascia is the fibrous connective tissue that binds skin to muscle, covers each muscle, and binds blood vessels and nerves together. Sometimes it forms tough, thick sheets, and sometimes it is quite thin and delicate. It separates, binds together, supports, and protects structures. It is composed of connective tissue fibers and cells and may contain fat.

Fascia of the body may be divided into two parts, superficial and deep. The superficial fascia of the body binds the skin to the deep fascia. It contains varying amounts of fat, usually more in women than men.

SUPERFICIAL FASCIA OF THE HEAD AND NECK

As already noted, the superficial fascia usually serves to bind the skin to the deep fascia. This is true of most of the superficial fascia of the head and neck. However, there is no deep fascia in the face and scalp where the muscles of facial expression are located. Instead, the superficial fascia is the site of attachment of the muscles of facial expression, and the skin is easily moved by these muscles.

DEEP FASCIA AND FASCIAL SPACES OF THE HEAD

The deep fascia of the head and neck begins at the nuchal and temporal lines and anterior border of the masseter muscle. It covers the muscles of mastication, is attached to the lower margin of the mandible, and ensheaths the neck.

A thick fascia covers the temporalis muscle. The temporal fascia separates from the muscle and attaches to the zygomatic arch (Figure 8-1).

The fascia around the masseter muscle envelopes the muscle and the parotid gland posterior to it. This fascia is called the parotideomasseteric fascia. It ends by blending with the fascia in front of the external auditory meatus and that over the mastoid process.

The medial pterygoid muscle is also covered by a tough fascia. The stylomandibular ligament blends with this fascia at the angle of the mandible.

Spaces exist between the muscles and between the fascia that cover and extend from them. The space between the temporalis fascia and the temporalis muscle includes part of the temporal fossa. This space is called the zygomaticotemporal space. The space between the medial pterygoid muscle and ramus of the mandible is called the pterygomandibular space. It is bounded above by the lateral pterygoid muscle and in front by the tendon of the temporalis. The space bounded by the parotideomasseteric fascia and the pterygoid fascia is called the masticator space. In addition, there is a space between the masseter and the buccinator muscle called the buccal space.

All of these spaces are filled to a greater or lesser degree with loose connective tissue containing fat. The fat is thinly encapsulated and is called the masticatory fat pad. The portion between the buccinator and masseter muscles is often called the buccal fat pad. While the spaces are separated from one another enough to warrant different names, they communicate with each other around fascial and muscular margins.

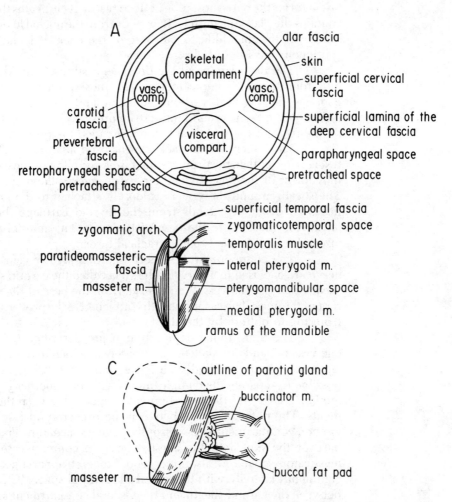

FIGURE 8–1 **(A) diagram of the fascae and compartments of the neck; (B) diagram of some of the fascial spaces in the face; (C) diagram of the buccal fat pad and surrounding space.**

DEEP FASCIA AND SPACES IN THE NECK

The neck may be thought of as a series of tubes within a tube. Its function is to support the head and, at the same time, allow for mobility of the head. The deep fascia in the neck compartmentalizes the skeleton, vessels, and viscera so that each of these elements can carry out its individual function while contributing to the function of the neck as a whole.

The deep fascia of the neck can be divided into superficial and deep portions or laminae. The superficial lamina of the deep cervical fascia forms the outermost tube of deep fascia. It ensheaths the neck and contains the platysma muscle. It extends from the nuchal lines and lower border of the mandible to the base of the neck. It is, however, not continuous but full of holes.

The deep lamina of the deep cervical fascia divides the neck into four tubular compartments. The most posterior compartment contains the cervical vertebral column and the anterior vertebral muscles. The fascia around these structures is very tough. The portion on the front of the vertebral column is called the prevertebral fascia.

The viscera of the neck are enclosed in a fascia. This visceral fascia is looser than the prevertebral fascia and allows for expansion and movement of the pharynx and larynx during swallowing and speech. The sheath around the viscera is loosely attached to the prevertebral fascia. In front, it extends from the thyroid cartilage, beneath the infrahyoid muscles, to the base of the neck. The anterior part of the visceral fascia is called the pretracheal fascia.

The common carotid artery, internal jugular vein, and vagus nerve are enclosed in a very tough fascia called the carotid sheath. The sheath encloses the vessels and nerve from the base of the skull to the root of the neck. The carotid sheath is attached to the prevertebral fascia from top to bottom by the alar fascia.

The four tubular compartments just described (two vascular, one visceral, and one skeletal) are loosely attached to one another, and any excess space is filled with loose connective tissue and fat. It is possible to separate the compartments from one another by blunt dissection. There are, therefore, potential spaces between the compartments. The potential space between the prevertebral fascia, and the visceral compartment is the retropharyngeal space. It extends from the base of the skull into the chest. Above, it communicates with the masticator space. At its upper end, the retropharyngeal space is continuous laterally with the lateral pharyngeal space. This space lies between the carotid sheath and the visceral compartment and extends inferiorly to where its name changes to the paravisceral space. It, too, is continuous above with the masticator space. The pretracheal space lies between the visceral compartment and the infrahyoid muscles. Like the retropharyngeal space, it extends into the chest. It is continuous laterally with the paravisceral space.

Virtually all of the potential spaces of the neck are in communication with each other and ultimately with the spaces around the muscles of mastication.

FLOOR OF THE MOUTH AND SUPRAHYOID REGION

The mylohyoid muscle forms the floor of the mouth. The potential space between the muscle and the oral mucosa is the sublingual space. The space can communicate with the suprahyoid area around the free margin of the mylohyoid muscle. The submandibular and submental fossae harbor potential spaces called the submandibular and submental spaces. They communicate with each other and with the masticator space.

FASCIAL SPACES AND THE SPREAD OF INFECTION

An abscess or other infection will spread by following the line of least resistance. Inflammation and the resulting pus may be confined to a limited area temporarily, but given enough time, the infection will fill a space and invade the nearest available one. Because of the extensive communications of the potential spaces, it is possible for an abscess of intraoral origin to extend all the way into the chest. An abscess from a maxillary molar tooth, for example, could invade the parotideomasseteric space. From there, it could enter the pterygomandibular space and then the retropharyngeal space. Within the retropharyngeal space, the infection could course downward to the chest. In actual practice, use of modern antibiotics and surgical techniques make it unlikely that such an extensive infection would occur. However, abscesses of dental origin involving one or more of the spaces described above are common.

Sometimes it is difficult to determine by inspection which tooth is responsible for the abscess. A few simple principles can narrow the field and aid in determining the offending tooth.

First, a spreading abscess always follows the course of least physical resistance. Periapical abscesses will invade the surrounding bone at its thinnest point and exit into the surrounding connective tissue. If a maxillary tooth is involved, the abscess will usually perforate on the buccal or labial side because the bone here is less dense than the bone of the palatal side of the tooth. However, if the root involved is very long or bent or if the bone is thinned by other pathological processes, the abscess will seek out the easiest exit.

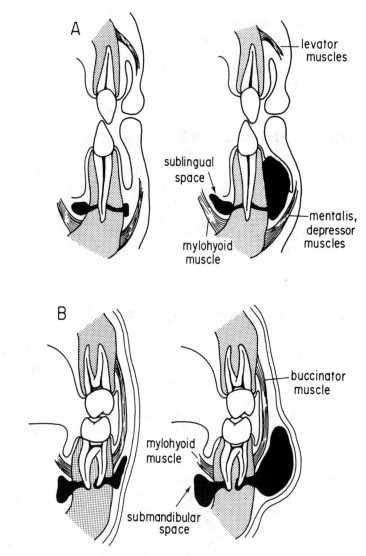

FIGURE 8–2   (A) diagram of the probable spread of an abscess in the mandibular incisive region; (B) diagram of the probable spread of a periapical abscess in the molar region.

In addition to the character of the bone, the location of muscle attachments affects the spread of infection. Muscle offers more resistance to penetration of an abscess than loose connective tissue. If an abscess perforates the labial or buccal side of the alveolar bone, it has two courses open to it. The abscess may grow and appear as a swelling in the labial or buccal vestibule, or it may penetrate the labial or buccal connective tissue and skin and appear on the face. Which course is taken partly depends upon whether or not the point of exit of the abscess is covered by a muscle attachment. In the incisive regions, the muscles are small and have little effect. Most abscesses here appear in the labial vestibule because the connective tissue is less dense and easier to penetrate. In the premolar region, however, the origins of the labial depressors below and elevators above are distal to the roots of the premolar teeth (Figure 8-2). An abscess from a premolar tooth would not penetrate the overlying muscle but would appear as a swelling in the vestibule. In contrast, in the molar region, the buccinator muscle is attached to the alveolar process well above the apices of the roots of the molar teeth (Figure 8-2). A periapical abscess from a molar tooth, which perforates the buccal side of the bone, will not be confined by the buccinator muscle and will be free to perforate the skin (Figure 8-2).

Finally, the mylohyoid muscle has the same effect on abscesses of mandibular teeth, which perforate the lingual alveolar bone (Figure 8-2). The mylohyoid is attached below the roots of all of the mandibular teeth except the third molars and sometimes the second molars. Lingual abscesses from the anterior six or seven teeth will swell and be confined to the sublingual space. Lingual abscesses from the third molar and sometimes second molar teeth will perforate below the attachment of the mylohyoid muscle and appear in the submandibular space.

CHAPTER SUMMARY

Fascia of the Head and Neck

Fascia	Location	Function or Special Features
Superficial	Face and scalp	Serves for attachment of muscles of facial expression
	Neck, occipital region, area under skin over muscles of mastication	Binds skin to deep fascia
Deep fascia of the head		
1. Temporal fascia	Over temporalis muscle	Attaches to the zygomatic arch
2. Parotideomasseteric fascia	Around masseter m. and parotid gland	
3. Pterygoid fascia	Covers pterygoid muscles	Blends with stylomandibular lig.
Deep fascia of the neck		
1. Superficial lamina	Ensheaths neck under superficial fascia	Contains platysma muscle, skin is attached to it by the superficial fascia
2. Deep lamina		
a. Prevertebral fascia	Surrounds the vertebral column and prevertebral muscles	
b. Visceral fascia	Surrounds the viscera of the neck	Anterior part is called the pretracheal fascia. Extends from the thyroid cartilage to the root of the neck.
c. Carotid sheath	Enclosed the carotid a., internal jugular v., and vagus n.	Extends from the base of the skull to the root of the neck
d. Alar fascia		Attaches the carotid sheath to the prevertebral fascia

Fascial Spaces of the Head and Neck

Space	Location	Communications
Zygomaticotemporal space	Between the temporalis fascia and the temporalis muscle	Masticator and pterygomandibular spaces
Pterygomandibular space	Between medial pterygoid muscle and the ramus of the mandible	Masticator space, lateral pharyngeal space, sublingual and submandibular spaces
Masticator space	Between the parotideomasseteric fascia and the pterygoid fascia	Lateral pharyngeal, sublingual and submandibular spaces
Buccal space	Between the masseter and buccinator muscles	Masticator space
Retropharyngeal space	Between the prevertebral fascia and the visceral fascia	Masticator space, lateral pharyngeal space
Lateral pharyngeal space	Between the carotid sheath and the visceral fascia, called the paravisceral space inferiorly	Masticator space, submandibular and retropharyngeal spaces
Pretracheal space	Between the visceral fascia and infrahyoid muscles	Extends to the chest, communicates with paravisceral space laterally
Sublingual space	Between the mylohyoid muscle and the oral mucosa	Submandibular and submental spaces
Submandibular space	In the submandibular fossa between the digastric m. and the body of the mandible	Masticator space, sublingual and submental spaces
Submental space	Between the anterior bellies of the digastric muscles and the mental symphysis	Masticator space, sublingual and submandibular spaces

STUDY EXERCISES

1. Where is the superficial fascia of the head and neck located? What is its function in the face and scalp? In the neck?

2. What is the location and function of the superficial lamina of the deep fascia of the neck?

3. The deep lamina of the deep fascia of the neck divides the neck into four compartments. Name these compartments and the portion of the deep lamina of the deep fascia of the neck that surrounds them.

4. *What is the function of the alar fascia?*

5. Name four spaces found in the head and neck.

6. *Give the location and communications of the spaces listed in Question 5.*

7. Why is it particularly important to manage infections that are located in spaces which communicate with the lateral pharyngeal space?

8. *Discuss the probable routes for the spread of periapical abscesses in incisor and molar teeth. If left unchecked, how many spaces could become involved in an infection which has entered the submandibular space?*

9

ANATOMIC
RELATIONSHIPS
AND DENTAL
ANESTHESIA

LEARNING OBJECTIVES

At the conclusion of this chapter, the student should be able to:

1. Describe some of the basic anatomic principles related to local dental anesthesia.
2. Describe the anatomy of regions most often involved in local dental anesthesia.

The purpose of this discussion is to review the structures and landmarks found in regions where local dental anesthesia might be administered. Before discussing each region, there are several anatomic facts of life which relate to injections in general. The student tends to think of bone as a dead substance rather than as living, sensitive tissue. All bones are covered by a connective tissue sheath, the periosteum. The periosteum is richly innervated. Touching or tearing it with a sharp object like a syringe needle will produce intense pain.

It is important not to inject a local anesthetic directly into an artery or vein. Because the vessels of the head and neck are extensively anastomosed and closely related to the brain and heart, neurologic and systemic reactions to injected substances can develop very rapidly. There is considerable variation in the position of blood vessels, especially veins. The pattern previously described is a generalization. While most major vessels like the carotid artery and internal jugular vein are relatively constant in location, the medium-sized and small branches are quite variable. The only way to be sure a syringe needle is not in a blood vessel is to aspirate with the syringe prior to injecting.

If a needle is inserted and then moved around, a considerable amount of damage can be done to blood vessels, resulting in a hematoma. Damage to vessels can also result in clotting within the vessel (thrombus). If a thrombus or a part of a thrombus then comes loose and travels into the vessels of the brain, the result will be a stroke. A needle should not be moved about excessively once inserted.

Finally, local anesthetics need not be injected into the nerve but only in the immediate vicinity. Inserting a needle directly into a nerve will cause intense pain and may damage the nerve. Also, nerves, like blood vessels, have a variable course and distribution so that the area anesthetized by a given injection may vary from person to person.

The regions of injection that will be discussed are the gingiva, the infratemporal fossa, the area around the mandibular foramen, the palate, and the region of the mental foramen.

THE GINGIVA

There are no large blood vessels or nerves in the gingiva. However, the gingiva is not very thick, and the alveolar bone beneath it is very sensitive as previously described.

THE INFRATEMPORAL FOSSA

The posterior superior alveolar nerves enter the maxillary bone above the maxillary tuberosity in the infratemporal fossa. Immediately behind the maxillary tuberosity are the pterygoid muscles and pterygoid venous plexus. Lateral to the maxilla are the buccal nerve and branches of the maxillary artery with accompanying veins. Medial to and above the back of the maxilla lies the pterygopalatine fossa and ganglion. The terminal branches of the maxillary artery enter the orbit and pterygopalatine fossa here. Anesthetic should be deposited near the foramina where the posterior superior alveolar nerves enter the maxillary bone. If the needle is pushed too far behind the maxilla or too far toward the pterygopalatine fossa, the risk of hematoma is increased. In addition, if anesthetic is allowed to enter the pterygopalatine fossa, the autonomic and some sensory innervation of the pharynx and soft palate will be interrupted, resulting in a very unpleasant sensation.

If the needle is inserted too far laterally or inferiorly, and anesthetic is injected, the posterior superior alveolar nerves will be unaffected, but some branches of the mandibular division of the trigeminal nerve may be deadened, particularly the buccal nerve.

THE MANDIBULAR REGION

The mandibular foramen is located approximately two centimeters behind the third molar and slightly below the occlusal plane. The anterior superior aspect is guarded by the lingula and attached sphenomandibular ligament. Below the opening is the attachment of the medial pterygoid muscle and part of the pterygoid venous plexus. The inferior alveolar nerve and vessels pass into the foramen from above and behind. The lingual nerve passes in front of the sphenomandibular ligament toward the tongue. The long buccal nerve passes anteriorly and laterally about one centimeter above the occlusal plane. It curves around the anterior edge of the mandibular ramus at a point in line with the notch of the lingula. The tendon of the temporalis muscle extends down along the anterior edge of the ramus beneath the buccal nerve. Anesthetic must be placed just above the lingular notch so that it will flow onto the inferior alveolar nerve.

A needle placed too far laterally will penetrate the temporalis tendon and may result in trismus and pain. Penetrating too far medially may result in the same problems with the medial pterygoid muscle. Injection below the back of the lingula will result in no anesthesia. Allowing the needle to travel too far posteriorly may result in damage to the inferior alveolar vessels and hematoma. Also deposition of anesthetic too far posterior to the lingular notch may cause drooping of the eyelid due to loss of innervation to the orbicularis oculi muscle.

The lingual nerve is so close to the inferior alveolar nerve that it is anesthetized at the same time. The long buccal nerve is usually anesthetized where it curves around the anterior margin of the mandibular ramus.

THE PALATE

The mucosa of the hard palate is firmly attached to the bone beneath. Since there is little submucosal space to accommodate a needle or anesthetic solution, this injection can be very uncomfortable to receive. The palatine vessels and nerves emerge from the greater palatine foramen medial to the maxillary third molar. The vessels and nerves lie in a groove with a little loose connective tissue. They run forward and communicate with the fellow of the opposite side. Also, the lesser palatine nerves supplying the soft palate should not be anesthetized as this creates a very unpleasant sensation.

The nasopalatine nerves emerge from the incisive foramen onto the front of the hard palate about one centimeter behind the central incisors. The right and left nerves emerge together and can be anesthetized with one injection. Care must be taken not to advance a needle through the incisive canal and into the nasal cavities.

THE INFRAORBITAL FORAMEN

The infraorbital foramen leads into the infraorbital canal and, therefore, into the orbit. There are no structures on the face that pose a hazard to injection, but the fact that the needle comes very close to the eyeball makes this site potentially very dangerous. The anterior and middle superior alveolar nerves can be deadened by injecting into the infraorbital canal.

THE MENTAL FORAMEN

The mental foramen is located about two centimeters below the occlusal plane between the bicuspids. It is shielded anteriorly by a small lip of bone and, therefore, must be approached from behind. The mental vessels emerge with the nerve and are to be avoided.

10

EMBRYOLOGY

LEARNING OBJECTIVES

At the conclusion of this chapter, the student should be able to:

1. Give a brief overview of the early embryology and formation of the three primary germ layers and the attainment of the general body form.
2. Know the fates of the germ layers.
3. Give the origin and fate of neural crest cells in the head and neck.
4. Discuss the development and fates of the pharyngeal arches, clefts, and pouches.
5. *Discuss the development of the tongue.*
6. Discuss the development of the face and nose.
7. Discuss the development of the palate, including the intermaxillary segment.
8. Describe the three stages of early tooth development.

This account is intended to acquaint the reader with the basic manner in which orally related structures of the head develop. To that end, the development of the germ layers, pharyngeal pouches, clefts, arches, maxillae, mandible, tongue, nose, face, palate, and teeth will be described.

GENERAL EMBRYOLOGY

Development of the Blastocyst

When the egg is ovulated, it enters the uterine tube and begins its journey toward the uterus. Fertilization takes place in the first part of the tube. The fertilized egg begins to divide into two-celled, four-celled, and eight-celled consecutive stages (Figure 10–1). When the developing egg reaches the uterus, four to five days after ovulation, it consists of a hollow ball of cells called the blastocyst. Inside the hollow ball is a small mass of cells stuck to one side called the inner cell mass. The inner cell mass will develop into the embryo, and the outer single cell layer of the blastocyst, called the trophoblast, will develop into the membranes and placenta.

The blastocyst embeds itself, inner cell mass end (embryonic pole) first, in the uterine wall (6–7 days post ovulation).

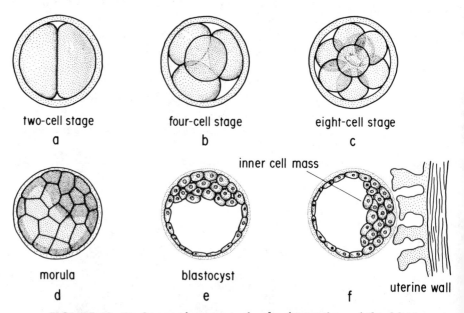

two-cell stage
a

four-cell stage
b

eight-cell stage
c

inner cell mass

morula
d

blastocyst
e

f

uterine wall

FIGURE 10–1 Successive stages in the formation of the blastocyst, from the two-celled stage (a) through the implanting blastocyst (f).

Formation of the Bilaminar Disc

The trophoblast at the embryonic pole of the blastocyst proliferates and produces a multinucleated layer without cell boundaries, the syncytio-trophoblast. The remainder of the trophoblast, which retains its mono-nucleate cellular character, is called the cytotrophoblast (Figure 10–2).

The inner cell mass also differentiates into two cell layers, the ectoderm and entoderm (Figure 10–2). The amniotic cavity is formed as a widening cleft between the ectoderm and cytotrophoblast. The roof of the new cavity becomes lined with cells called amnioblasts, which are probably derived from the cytotrophoblast.

The blastocyst becomes lined with small, flattened cells pro-duced by the cytotrophoblast. The cells remain attached to each other but detach (delaminate) from the cytotrophoblast, delimiting a cavity within the blastocyst called the primary yolk sac. The roof of the primary yolk sac is the layer of entoderm (Figure 10–2). The space between the primary yolk sac and the trophoblast is filled with a loose, connective-tissue-like material called extraembryonic mesoderm. It is produced by the cytotrophoblast (Figure 10–2).

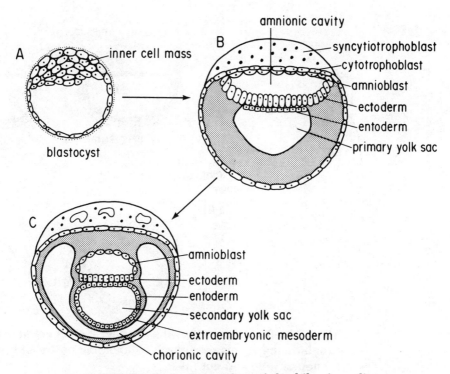

FIGURE 10–2   Formation of the bilaminar disc.

All this time, the trophoblast is enlarging, and the developing blastocyst is becoming deeply embedded in the uterine wall. The trophoblast enlarges faster than the embryo so that spaces develop in the extraembryonic mesoderm. The spaces coalesce into a large cavity, the chorionic cavity (Figure 10-2). The extraembryonic mesoderm forms a layer covering the embryo, primitive yolk sac, and amnionic cavity and lining the chorionic cavity. The embryo remains attached to the trophoblast by mesoderm. This attachment is called the connecting stalk. It is the future umbilical cord.

The entoderm proliferates and lines the inside of the primary yolk sac, which is then called the secondary yolk sac (Figure 10-2). The developing embryo is now a disc consisting of a layer of ectoderm and a layer of entoderm and is said to be bilaminar.

The bilaminar disc is flat with an egg-shaped outline (Figure 10-3). The future head end is wider than the future anal end. The ectoderm and entoderm of the disc become very firmly adherent at two areas. One such area, the prochordal plate, is located at the head end of the embryo and will become the oral opening. The other area, the cloacal plate, is at the opposite end of the embryo and will be the anal and urogenic openings.

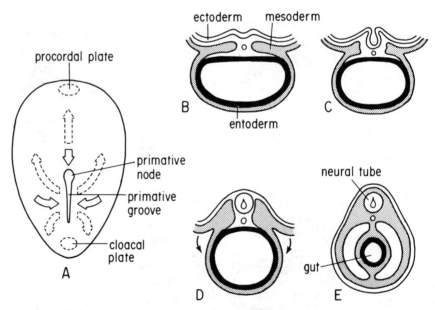

FIGURE 10–3   Diagram showing the migration of ectodermal cells to form intraembryonic mesoderm (A). Folding of the embryo to form the neural tube and gut (B–E).

Formation of the Trilaminar Disc

The extraembryonic mesoderm, as the name implies, lies outside the embryo. This mesoderm does not take part in forming any part of the embryo. The formation of intraembryonic mesoderm results in an embryo with three germ layers, the trilaminar disc. Intraembryonic mesoderm arises in the following manner.

During the third week of development, the primitive streak or groove appears in the midline toward the anal end of the embryo (Figure 10–3). The streak becomes more prominent, ending cephalically in an elevated area, called the primitive node, which surrounds a small pit. Cells from the ectodermal layer begin to move into the groove and spread out between the surface ectodermal layer and the underlying entodermal layer. This new layer of cells between the ectoderm and entoderm is the intraembryonic mesoderm or, simply, the mesodermal germ layer. Some cells of the ectodermal layer invaginate through the pit at the primitive node and turn immediately forward. These cells form the notochord.

More and more cells migrate through the groove and spread out laterally. The mesoderm eventually reaches the edge of the embryonic disc and merges with the extraembryonic mesoderm (Figure 10–3). Mesoderm cannot migrate between the ectoderm and entoderm of the prochordal plate or cloacal plate.

Formation of the Neural Tube and Gut

By the end of the third week of development, the embryo consists of three primary germ layers and is ready to begin developing organ systems. Through a system of folding and fusion, two tubes are formed—the neural tube and the gut. The neural tube will give rise to the brain and spinal cord. The gut will become the alimentary system.

The Neural Tube. The ectoderm thickens, and a distinct, slipper-shaped plate, the neural plate, forms. The lateral edges, or neural folds, meet at the midline and form the neural tube (Figures 10–3 and 10–4). At the cephalic end, the neural tube undergoes very complex alterations to become the brain. The remainder of the tube becomes the spinal cord. Specialized cells located on the crests of the neural folds separate from them and occupy a position lateral to the neural tube (Figure 10–4). These neural crest cells develop into the dorsal root ganglia and cranial sensory ganglia. In the head, these cells also migrate and give rise to all mesodermal structures except the skeletal muscles.

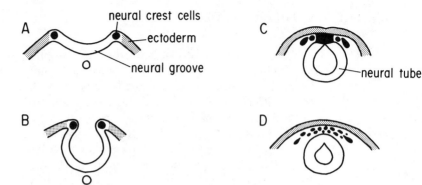

FIGURE 10-4   Closure of the neural tube and origin of neural crest cells.

The Gut.   While the neural tube is forming by upward folding of the ectoderm, the gut is formed by downward folding of the edges of the ectoderm and mesoderm (Figure 10-3). The edges of the former embryonic disc fold downward on the yolk sac. Most of the yolk sac is covered by extraembryonic mesoderm. As the folding continues, the portion of the yolk sac covered by extraembryonic mesoderm is pinched off, and a new tube is formed by the fusion of the folds at the ventral midline. The embryo now has a ventral tube extending from the prochordal plate to the cloacal plate. This tube is lined with entoderm and covered with mesoderm. The entire external surface of the embryo is covered with ectoderm.

Fates of the Germ Layers

Each germ layer gives rise to certain tissues and organs. Ectoderm gives rise mainly to structures that communicate with the environment: the central nervous system; the peripheral nervous system; sensory epithelia of the eye, ear, and nose; the epidermis, hair, and nails; the glands of the skin; the mammary glands; the pituitary gland; dental enamel; and the lining of the oral cavity.

The mesodermal germ layer gives rise to connective tissue; cartilage and bone; muscle; dermis of the skin; kidneys; membranes that line the peritoneal, pleural, and pericardial cavities; blood; blood vessels; heart; and spleen.

Entoderm gives rise to structures associated with the gut: the lining of the gut; the parenchyma of the tonsil, the thyroid, the parathyroids; the thymus; the liver and pancreas; the lining of the respiratory system; the lining of the urinary bladder and urethra; the lining of the tympanic cavity; and the Eustachian tubes.

It should be repeated that, in the head, neural crest cells give rise to all mesodermal structures (smooth muscle, cartilage, bone, general connective tissue) except skeletal (striated) muscle.

Development of Pharyngeal Arches, Clefts, and Pouches

With the closure of the neural tube and gut comes the beginning of the development of external body form. The entire outside of the embryo is covered with ectoderm and is bent in the craniocaudal direction. This bending results in movement of the prochordal plate to beneath the developing brain where the mouth will be. The prochordal plate is now called the buccopharyngeal membrane. Its ectodermal side faces outward, and its entodermal side is inside. The head end of the gut tube, the foregut, is just inside the buccopharyngeal membrane. The depression outside of the buccopharyngeal membrane is the stomodeum, or future mouth. The oral cavity is formed by deepening (invagination) of the ectodermally lined stomodeum. The buccopharyngeal membrane moves inward as the oral cavity deepens and eventually stops at the level of the oral pharyngeal isthmus. The ectodermally lined oral cavity and entodermally lined foregut become continuous when the buccopharyngeal membrane ruptures and disappears.

If a four-week-old embryo is viewed face on (Figure 10-5), the stomodeum is seen to occupy the center of the developing face. The brain bulges above it with bilateral nasal placodes. The developing heart bulges below the stomodeum.

During the fourth and fifth weeks, five outpocketings of the foregut develop (Figure 10-5). They are lined with entoderm and protrude into the wall of the prospective pharynx. They are called the pharyngeal pouches. At the same time, four clefts appear on the outside of the embryo. These pharyngeal clefts are ectodermally lined invaginations of the external surface. The clefts and pouches deepen and approach each other but do not normally become continuous. The clefts and pouches divide the tissue of the pharyngeal region into bars, called pharyngeal arches (Figure 10-5). There are six arches but the fifth is transient.

Fates of the Pharyngeal Arches

The external surface of each pharyngeal arch is covered with ectoderm, while the internal surface is covered with entoderm. The center of each arch consists of mesoderm containing a bar of cartilage and a nerve. Therefore, considering the fates of the pharyngeal arches entails: (1) defining the muscles that develop from the mesoderm of each arch; (2) determining the structures that develop from the cartilage of each arch; and (3) naming the cranial nerve that is associated with each arch.

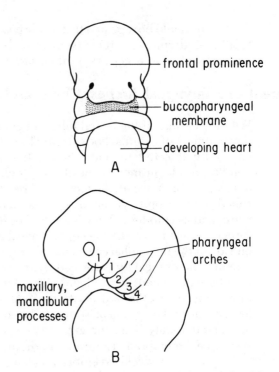

FIGURE 10–5   (A) anterior view of a four-week-old embryo; (B) lateral view of a five-week-old embryo showing pharyngeal arches 1 through 4.

The first arch is called the mandibular arch. It divides into two parts, the maxillary process and the mandibular process. The muscles of mastication develop from the mesoderm of the first arch. The cartilage of the maxillary process disappears, but parts of the cartilage of the mandibular process, Meckel's cartilage, persist. A portion of Meckel's cartilage becomes fibrous and is called the sphenomandibular ligament. The dorsal ends of cartilage become the malleus and incus bones of the middle ear. The fifth cranial nerve is the nerve of the first arch.

The second arch is called the hyoid arch. The muscles derived from this arch are the muscles of facial expression, the posterior belly of the digastric, the stylohyoid, and the auricular muscles. The nerve of the second arch is the facial (VII). The cartilage of the second arch is called Reichert's cartilage and gives rise to the stapes, the styloid process, the stylohyoid ligament, and parts of the hyoid bone.

Muscles derived from the third pharyngeal arch are the stylopharyngeus and superior pharyngeal constrictor. The cartilage of the third arch forms part of the body and greater horns of the hyoid bone. The nerve of the third arch is the glossopharyngeal.

The fourth and sixth arches are difficult to separate. The muscles derived from these arches are the pharyngeal constrictors and some of the laryngeal muscles. The cartilages fuse to form the thyroid, cricoid, and laryngeal cartilages. The nerves are the vagus and spinal accessory nerves.

Fates of the Pharyngeal Clefts

The fates of the pharyngeal clefts are quite uncomplicated. The first cleft forms the external auditory canal. The inferior edge of the second pharyngeal arch proliferates and extends inferiorly to cover, and eventually obliterate, the remaining clefts. Occasionally, a cleft will persist as a space called a cervical sinus or cyst (Figure 10-6).

Fates of the Pharyngeal Pouches

The entodermally lined pharyngeal pouches have a slightly more complex fate than the clefts. The first pouch becomes the Eustachian tube. The entoderm of the second pouch becomes the palatine tonsil. The inferior parathyroid glands and thymus develop from the third pouch. The fourth pouch gives rise to the superior parathyroids, and the entoderm of the fifth pouch produces the ultimobranchial body, which becomes the parafollicular cells of the thyroid gland.

Development of the Tongue, Face, Nose, and Palate

Although the tongue, face, nose, and palate will be considered separately, they all form at the same time, beginning at about the fourth week of development.

Development of the Tongue. The tongue begins as two lateral lingual swellings and one medial swelling, the tuberculum impar, in the floor of the oral cavity. The swellings are the result of proliferation of the mesoderm of the mandibular process of the first pharyngeal arch. Another medial swelling, the hypobranchial eminence, forms just posterior to the tuberculum impar and is derived from the mesoderm of the second, third, and part of the fourth arches. The lateral lingual swellings enlarge and overgrow the tuberculum impar. They fuse to form the anterior two thirds or body of the tongue. The root of the tongue is formed by proliferation of the third arch over the hypobranchial eminence. The epiglottis develops from the fourth arch.

Development of the Face and Nose. At four weeks of development, the face consists of a median bulge, called the frontal prominence, and the maxillary and mandibular processes of the first

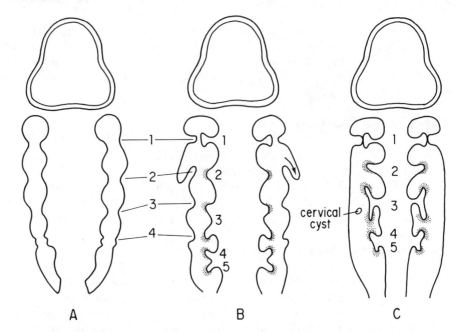

FIGURE 10-6 Successive stages in the development of the pharyngeal pouches and clefts. Pouches are numbered on the inside, and clefts are numbered on the outside.

arch. At about four and one half weeks, bilateral thickenings appear in the ectoderm just above the lateral margins of the stomodeum. These are the nasal placodes or future olfactory epithelia. The placodes begin to invaginate to form the nasal pits. At five weeks, the mesoderm surrounding the nasal pits proliferates and forms the medial and lateral nasal swellings. The eyes appear on the lateral aspect of the head. The future nasolacrimal duct appears as a groove extending from the eye to the lateral nasal swelling (Figure 10-7).

The face is formed by proliferation, removal, and fusion of mesoderm of various processes and swellings. Lateral swellings and processes move medially, compressing tissue between them.

About the sixth and seventh weeks of development, the maxillary processes and lateral nasal swellings move toward the midline (Figure 10-8). The nasal pits and swellings are pushed closer together as they are moved toward the midline (Figure 10-8). The lateral nasal swellings will become the alar part of the nose. The medial nasal swellings merge toward the midline as the maxillary processes continue to grow toward each other. The medial nasal swellings form the center of the upper lip. The maxillary processes fuse with this central portion to form the lateral portions of the upper lip (Figure 10-8). The

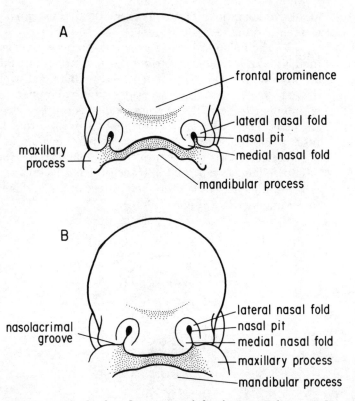

FIGURE 10–7   Early development of the face: (A) five weeks, (B) six weeks.

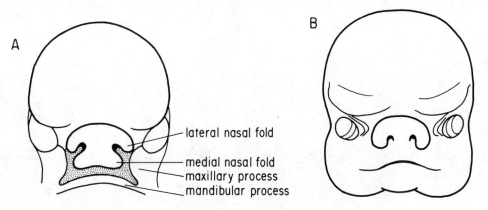

FIGURE 10–8   Later development of the face: (A) seven weeks, (B) ten weeks.

nasolacrimal groove closes to form the nasolacrimal duct, and the elements of the face are complete.

The palate is being formed at the same time as the face. The medial nasal swellings contribute to more than just the upper lip. In addition to this labial component, the medial nasal swellings merge at deeper levels to form an upper jaw component and a palatal component. These three components comprise the intermaxillary segment. The upper jaw component carries the four incisor teeth. It fuses with the maxillary bones, which develop in the maxillary processes of each side to complete the dental arch. From each medial nasal swelling, a small shelf of tissue projects backward from the upper jaw component. These little shelves fuse at the midline and are called the primary palate (Figure 10-9).

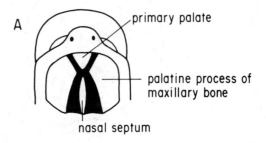

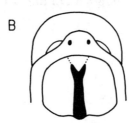

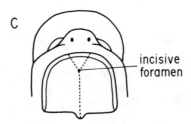

FIGURE 10-9 Successive stages of closure of the palate.

At the same time, the tongue appears in the floor of the mouth. The nasal pits have deepened and widened to form the primitive nasal cavities. A septum remains between the cavities, but they have no floor and communicate with the oral cavity (Figure 10-10). This communication will be closed by formation of the secondary palate. The secondary palate begins as bilateral shelf-like projections from the maxillary bones. Initially, each shelf of the secondary palate projects downward on either side of the developing tongue. As development proceeds, the shelves lift upward and meet at the midline. They fuse with each other, with the nasal septum, and with the primary palate (Figures 10-9 and 10-10). The incisive foramen marks the anterior end of the palatal raphe.

Occasionally, during development of the face and palate, one or more structures fail to fuse, resulting in clefts. A cleft may be unilateral or bilateral. It may involve the lip, primary palate, secondary palate, or any combination of the three. Rarely, the nasolacrimal duct

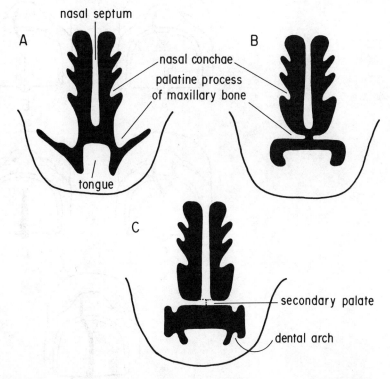

FIGURE 10–10 Frontal section of the nasal and oral cavities of a embryo to show closure of the palate: (A) seven weeks, (B) eight weeks, (C) ten weeks.

fails to form properly, resulting in a facial cleft extending from the medial corner of the eye to the nose or upper lip. Cleft lip and cleft of the primary palate usually occur between the medial nasal process and the maxillary process and the primary and secondary palates respectively. A midline cleft of the lip or primary palate is extremely rare but does occur. The more common clefts are illustrated in Figure 10–11.

The mandible develops within the mandibular process of the first pharyngeal arch. The cartilage of the mandibular process, Meckel's cartilage, marks the course of the mandibular canal. It does not contribute to the bony mandible but disappears as previously described. The mandible develops in halves from mesodermal tissues and cartilages of the first arch. Each half of the body and each ramus join separate coronoid and condylar cartilages. The two halves then merge at the mental symphysis with a mental cartilage. The alveolar process of the mandible is a separate bone that develops in response to the devel-

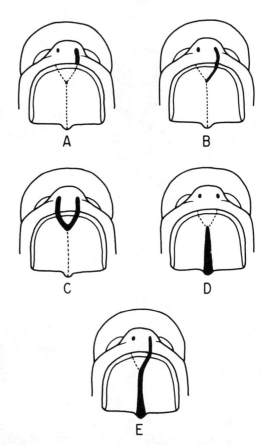

FIGURE 10–11 Common clefts of the lip and palate.

oping teeth. It fuses with the body of the mandible but will be reabsorbed if a tooth is lost.

The mandible grows by lengthening of the condylar neck and by adding bone to the back of the ramus while removing it from the front.

Development of the Teeth

A thickening in the oral ectoderm along the line of the future arches appears at about six weeks of development. This thickening is called the dental lamina. Early tooth development takes place in three stages: the bud stage, the cap stage, and the bell stage. Cells of the dental lamina proliferate at the site of each future tooth in the dental arch. The cells form a small knot or bud, which projects into the underlying mesoderm. The tooth is said to be in the bud stage (Figure 10-12). The bud invaginates on its deep surface forming a double-walled, cap-shaped enamel organ. The enamel organ will produce the enamel of the tooth. The developing tooth is now said to be in the cap stage (Figure 10-12).

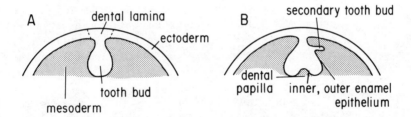

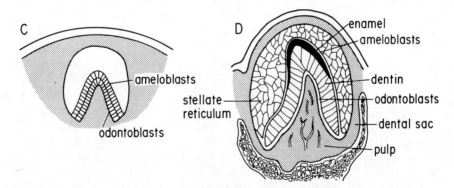

FIGURE 10-12   Stages of tooth development: (A) bud stage, (B) cap stage, (C) early bell stage, (D) late bell stage.

It is still attached to the dental lamina. The mesoderm under the cap proliferates and organizes into a small knob of tissue called the dental papilla (Figure 10–12). The dental papilla will give rise to the dental pulp and odontoblasts and thus dentin.

During the bell stage, the enamel organ differentiates further. It elongates and surrounds the papilla, taking on a bell shape (Figure 10–12). The cells of the enamel organ that are apposed closely to the papilla are called the inner enamel epithelium. The cells that form the outside of the "bell" are called the outer enamel epithelium. The space between the inner and outer enamel epithelium is filled with a loose network of cells called the stellate reticulum.

The dental papilla undergoes further development. A general proliferation of papilla cells occurs. Cells nearest the inner enamel epithelium differentiate and form a single layer of cells, the odonto-blasts. The odontoblasts will produce dentin. In addition, connective tissue around the developing tooth thickens. This is the beginning of the dental sac. The dental sac will give rise to the periodontal fibers, cementoblasts, and alveolar bone.

The odontoblasts of the dental papilla induce the cells of the inner enamel epithelium to become ameloblasts, or enamel-producing cells. The odontoblasts begin making dentin at the tip of the future crown of the tooth. The ameloblasts wait for the first layer of dentin to be laid down, and then they begin producing enamel over the new dentin. As the odontoblasts produce layers of dentin, the pulp cavity becomes smaller. Also, as the ameloblasts produce more enamel, the stellate reticulum is reduced.

When the crown of the tooth is complete, root formation begins. At the future cementoenamel junction, the inner and outer enamel epithelia become apposed. The new structure is called the epithelial root sheath of Hertwig. The root sheath extends past the base of the developing tooth and induces odontoblasts along the surface of the future root. The root sheath forms a diaphragm across the bottom of the tooth, leaving a hole called the apical canal. No ameloblasts are formed. As soon as a layer of dentin is deposited, the root sheath in that area breaks down, and the new dentin comes into contact with the cells of the dental sac. Cementoblasts differentiate from the dental sac and begin producing cementum. Periodontal fibers become embedded in the cementum and the developing alveolar bone.

The means by which the size and shape of a tooth are controlled is unknown. A small primordium of the secondary tooth develops from the dental lamina lingual to the enamel organ of each deciduous tooth between the fifth month *in utero* and ten months of age. The dental lamina extends distal to the enamel organ of the second deciduous molar and premordia of the third molars are formed. Secondary teeth develop exactly like the primary teeth.

CHAPTER SUMMARY

Fates of the Germ Layers

Germ Layer	Fate
Ectoderm	1. Central nervous system 2. Peripheral nervous system 3. Epidermis 4. Hair and nails 5. Glands of the skin 6. Enamel of the teeth 7. Lining of the oral cavity 8. *Sensory epithelium of the ear and eye* 9. *Mammary glands* 10. *Neurohypophysis of pituitary gland*
Mesoderm	1. Connective tissue 2. Cartilage 3. Bone 4. Muscle 5. Dermis of the skin 6. *Kidneys* 7. *Membranes that line the peritoneal, pleural, and pericardial cavities* 8. *Blood, blood vessels, and heart* 9. *Spleen*
Entoderm (Endoderm)	1. Lining of the gut 2. *Parenchyma of the tonsils, thyroid, and parathyroids, thymus, liver, and pancreas* 3. *Lining of the respiratory system* 4. *Lining of the urinary bladder and urethra* 5. *Lining of the tympanic cavity and Eustachian tube*
Neural crest cells	All mesodermal structures in the head except striated muscle

continued on the following page

Fates of the Pharyngeal Arches

Arch	Muscle	Cartilage	Nerve
1st (Mandibular arch)	Muscles of mastication	Meckel's cartilage; Malleus, incus, sphenomandibular ligament	V
2nd (Hyoid arch)	1. Muscles of facial exp. 2. Post. belly of the digastric muscle 3. Stylohyoid muscle 4. Auricular muscles	Reichert's cartilage; 1. Stapes 2. Styloid process 3. Stylohyoid ligament 4. Part of the hyoid bone	VII
3rd	1. Stylopharyngeus m. 2. Sup. pharyngeal constrictor m.	Body and greater horns of the hyoid	IX
4th and 6th	1. Pharyngeal constrictor muscles 2. Laryngeal muscles	Thyroid, cricoid, and laryngeal cartilages	X and XI
5th arch is transient			

Fates of the Pharyngeal Pouches

Pouch	Fate
1st	Becomes Eustachian tube
2nd	Becomes palatine tonsil
3rd	Becomes inferior parathyroid glands and thymus
4th	Forms superior parathyroid glands
5th	Forms the ultimobranchial body (UB) (parafollicular cells of the thyroid gland)

Early Tooth Development

Stage	Developing Structures	Fates or Functions of Structures
Bud stage	Dental lamina	Cells of the lamina proliferate and produce a small knot or bud.
Cap stage	The bud invaginates on its deep side, forming a double-walled, cap-shaped enamel organ. The dental papilla forms from the mesoderm under the "cap".	The enamel organ will produce the enamel of the tooth. The dental papilla will give rise to the dental pulp, odontoblasts, and thus, dentin.
Bell stage	The enamel organ differentiates, elongates, and surrounds the dental papilla. The dental papilla differentiates, forming odontoblasts; dental sac forms.	Inner and outer enamel epithelia and stellate reticulum form. Odontoblasts produce dentin. The dental sac gives rise to periodontal fibers, cementoblasts, and alveolar bone.

STUDY EXERCISES

1. What is the bilaminar disc? What is the trilaminar disc?

2. Name the three primary germ layers. What role do neural crest cells have in the head and neck?

3. List the fates of each of the primary germ layers.

4. What is a pharyngeal arch? *Describe the arrangement of the three primary germ layers in the pharyngeal arch. List each arch, its associated nerve, and the fate of its cartilaginous and muscular component.*

5. What is a pharyngeal pouch? List the fates of each pharyngeal pouch.

6. What is a pharyngeal cleft? What are the fates of the clefts?

7. *The tongue develops from the proliferation of which germ layer from which arches?*

8. The maxillary and mandibular processes both develop from which arch?

9. Name the two folds around the nasal pits.

10. What is the intermaxillary segment? Name the three things which form from it.

11. What is the primary palate? The secondary palate? *How do they differ in embryonic origin?*

12. *List some of the more common clefts of the lip and/or palate and the structures that fail to fuse, thus producing the cleft.*

13. List the three stages of early tooth development. Under each stage, list the structures that appear, and briefly describe the function of each structure.

14. Does the alveolar bone of each dental arch develop if the teeth do not develop?

REFERENCES

Arey, Leslie Brainard. *Developmental Anatomy*. W.B. Saunders Co., Philadelphia, 1974.

Bloom, William and Don W. Fawcett. *A Textbook of Histology*. 10th ed., W.B. Saunders, Co., Philadelphia, 1975.

Du Brul, Lloyd E. *Sicher's Oral Anatomy*. 7th ed., C.V. Mosby Co., St. Louis, 1980.

Fried, Lawrence A. *Anatomy of the Head, Neck, Face, and Jaws*. Lea and Febiger, 1976.

Guyton, Arthur C. *Textbook of Medical Physiology*. 5th ed., W.B. Saunders Co., Philadelphia, 1976.

Gray, Henry. *Gray's Anatomy*. Roger Warwick and Peter L. Williams, eds., W.B. Saunders Co., Philadelphia, 1973.

Langman, Jan. *Medical Embryology*. William and Wilkins Co., Baltimore, 1975.

Manter and Gatz's Essentials of Clinical Neuroanatomy and Neurophysiology. Ronald G. Clark, ed., F.A. Davis Co., Philadelphia, 1975.

Project Acorde. Department of Health, Education, and Welfare. *Administration of Local Anesthetic*. Quercus Corp., Castro Valley, Calif., 1976.

Snell, Richard S. *Clinical Anatomy for Medical Students*. Little Brown and Co., Boston, 1973.

Sperber, Geoffrey H. *Craniofacial Embryology*. John Wright and Sons, Ltd., Distributed by Year Book Medical Publishers, Chicago, 1975.

Woodburne, Russel T. *Essentials of Human Anatomy*. Oxford University Press, New York, 1961.

SELECTED FIGURES
FOR STUDY

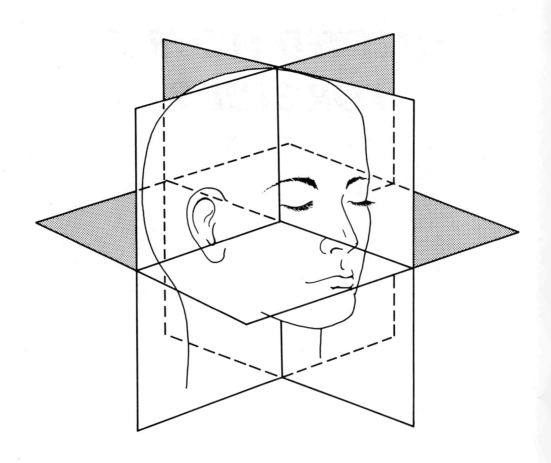

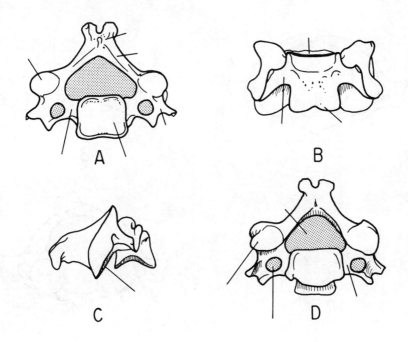

A

B

C

D

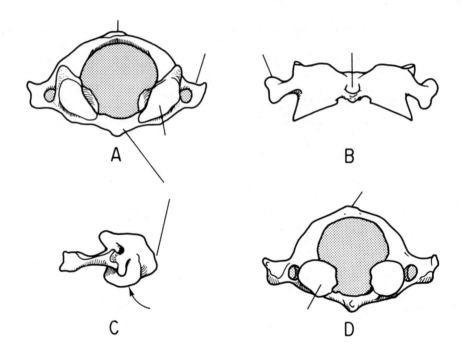

A

B

C

D

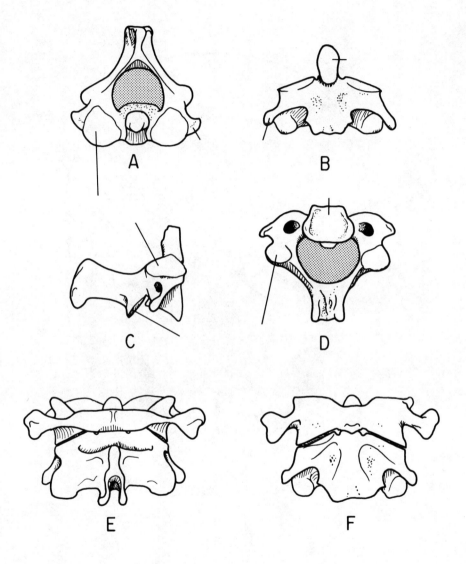

A

B

C

D

E

F

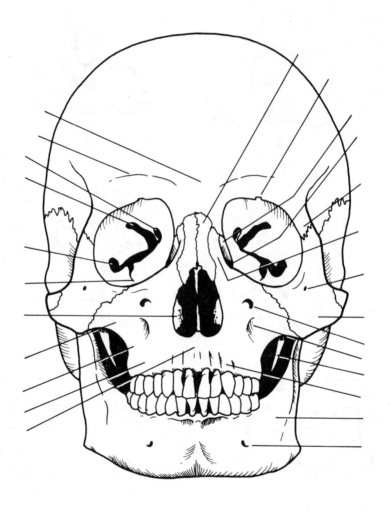

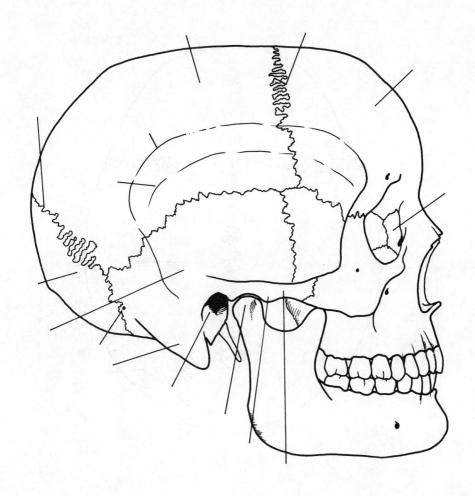

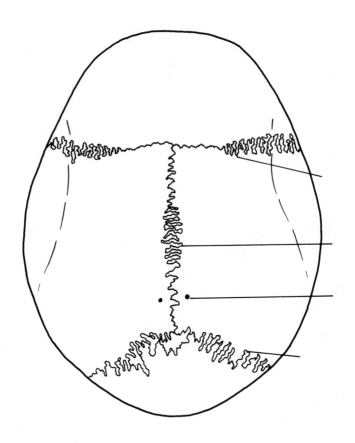

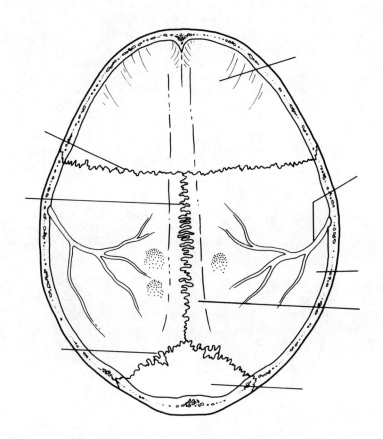

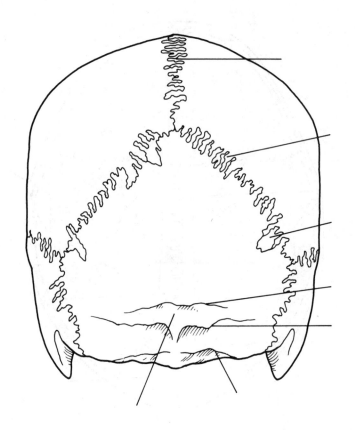

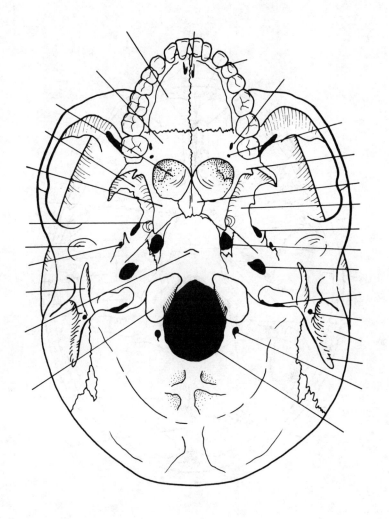

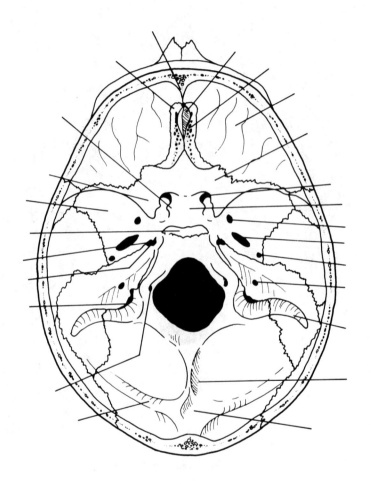

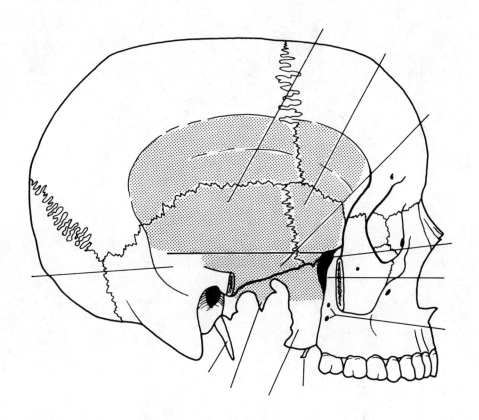

A

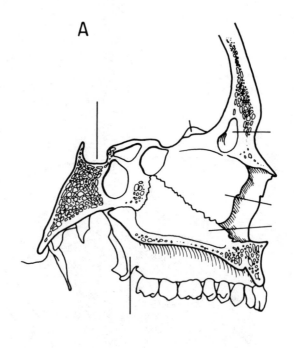

B

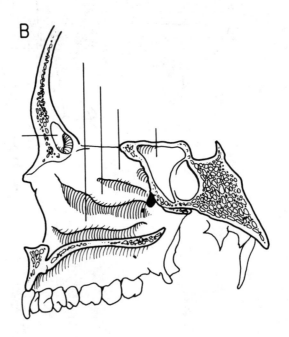

186

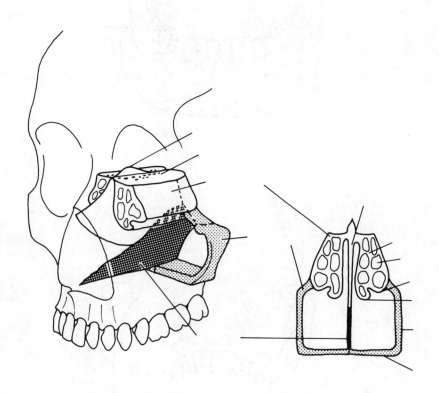

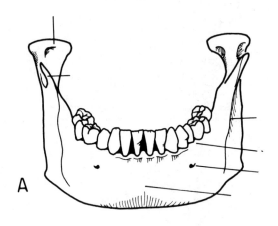

A

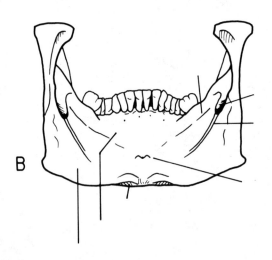

B

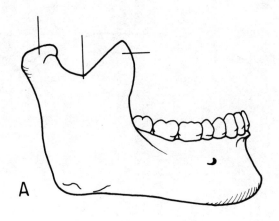

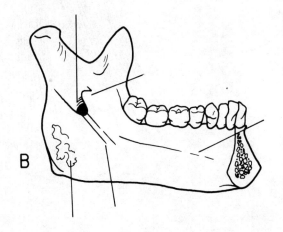

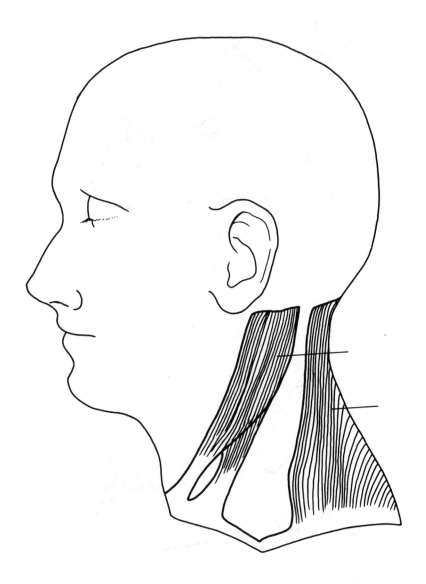

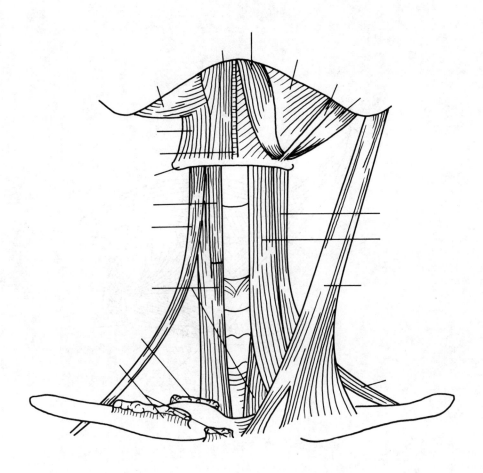

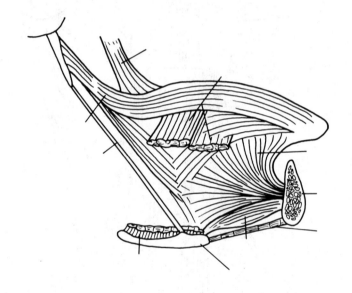

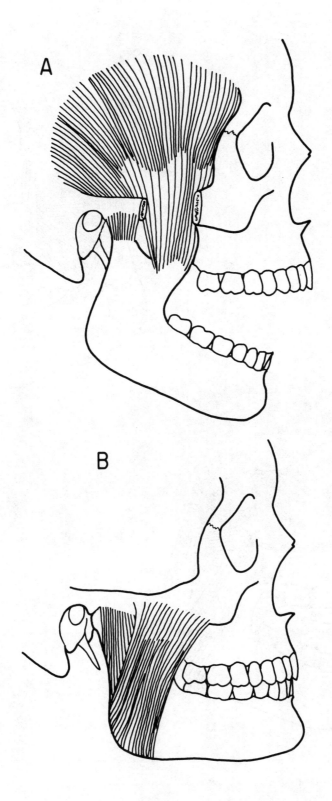

A

B

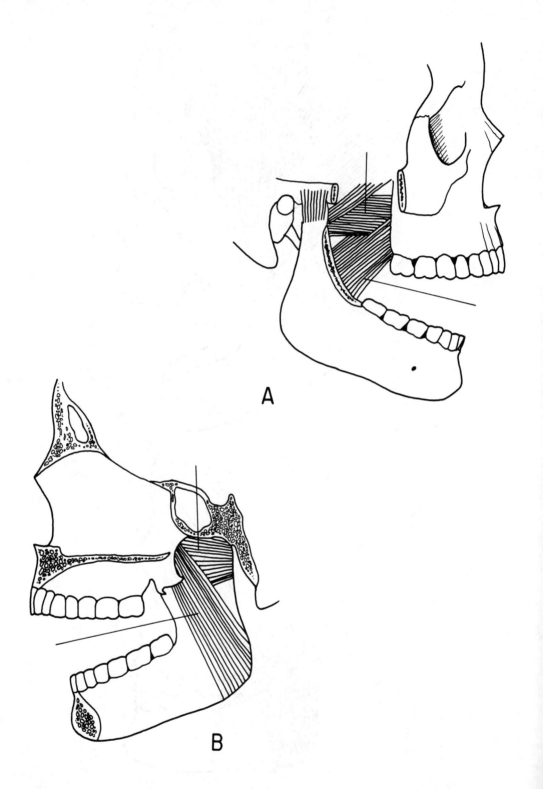

A

B

194

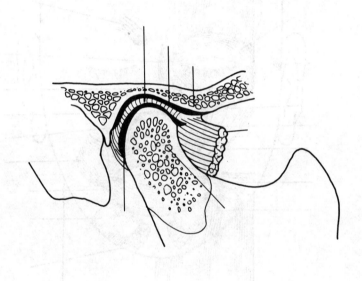

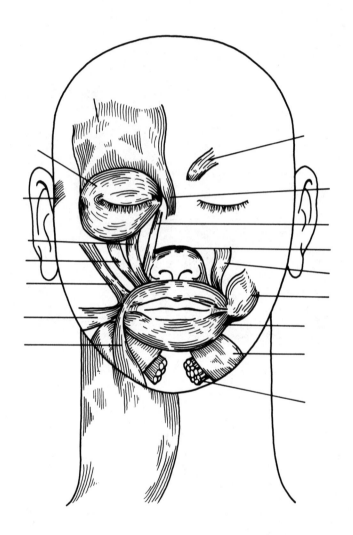

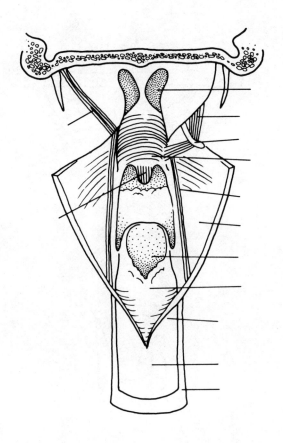

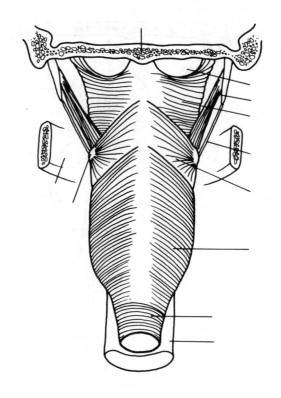

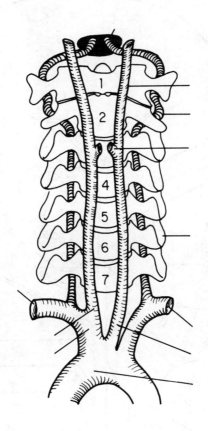

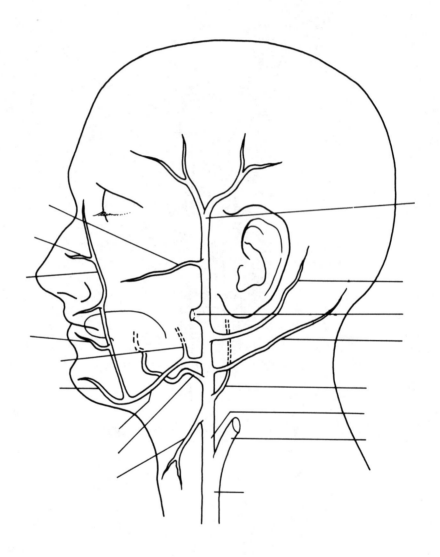

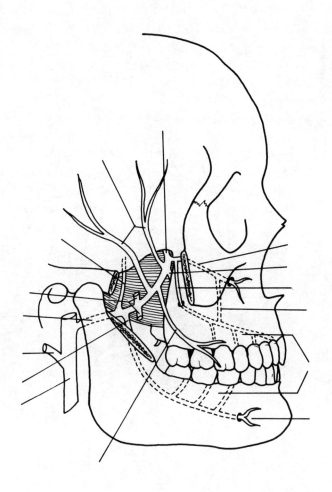

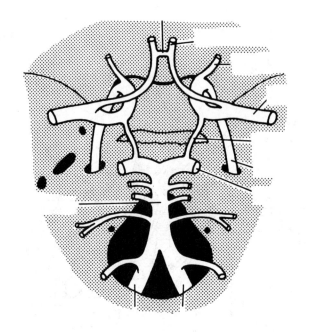

202

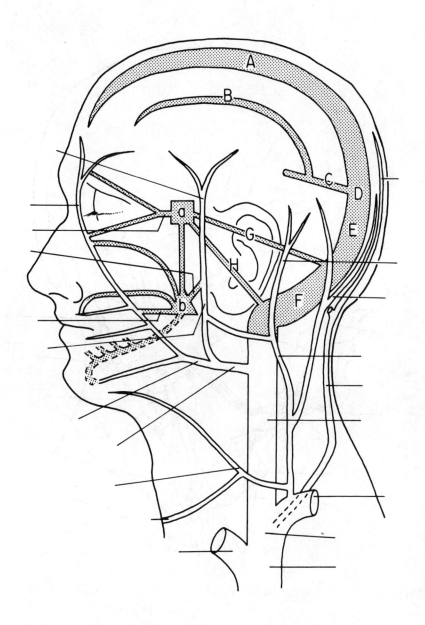

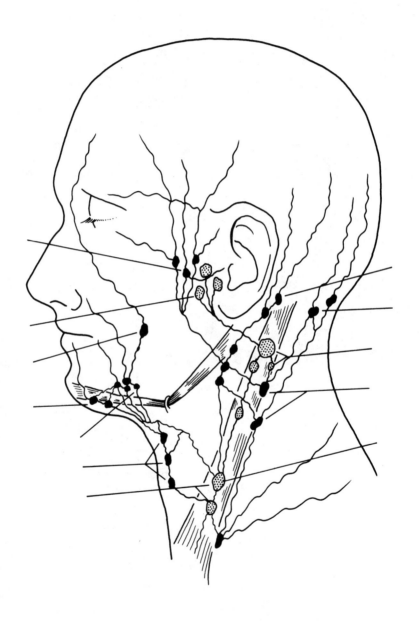

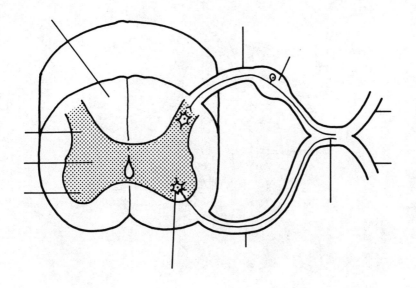

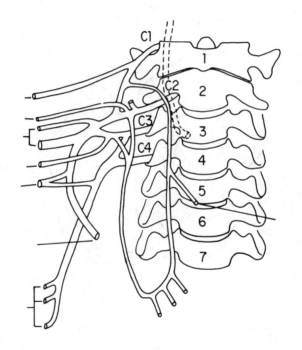

C1
1
C2
2
C3
3
C4
4
5
6
7

206

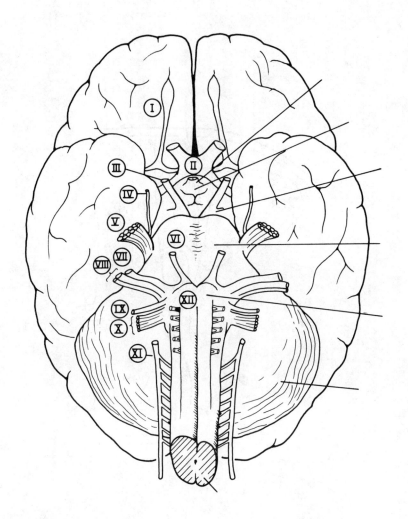

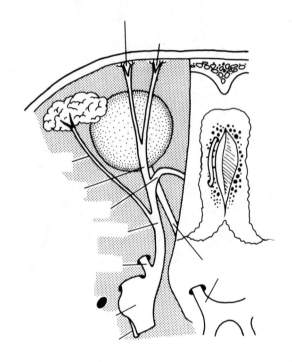

208

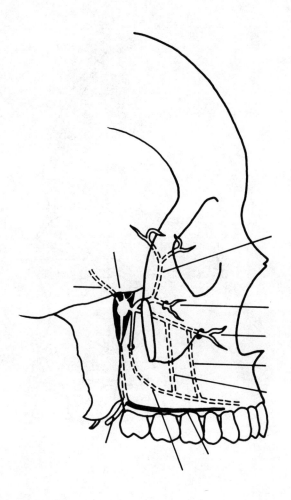

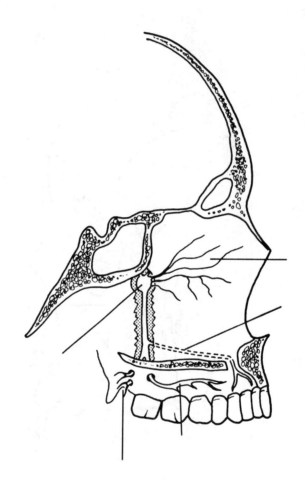

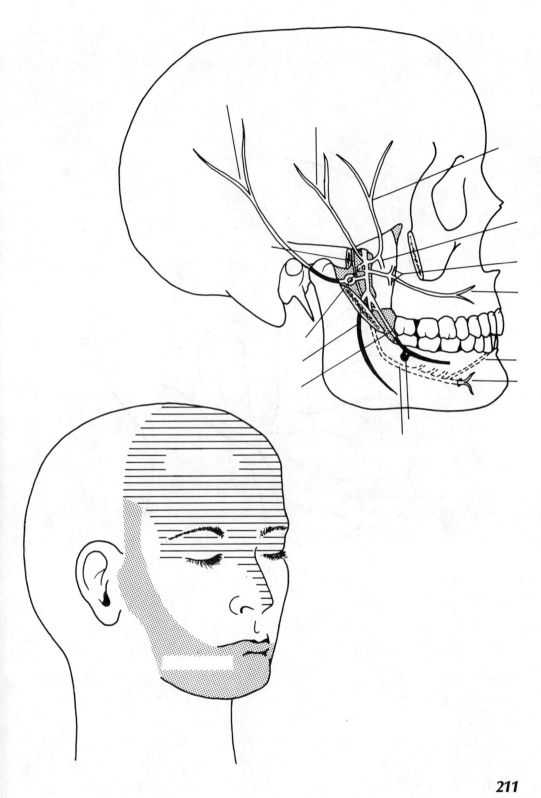

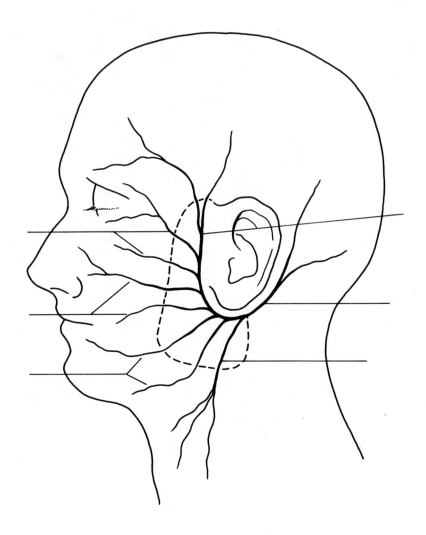

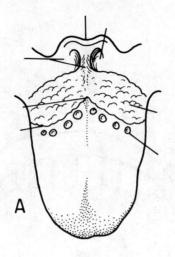

A

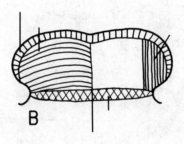

B

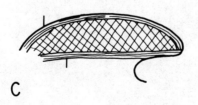

C

213

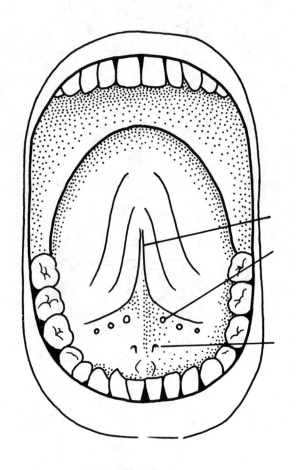

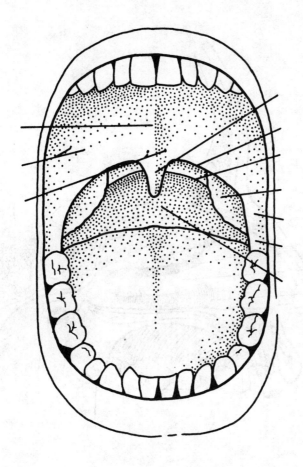

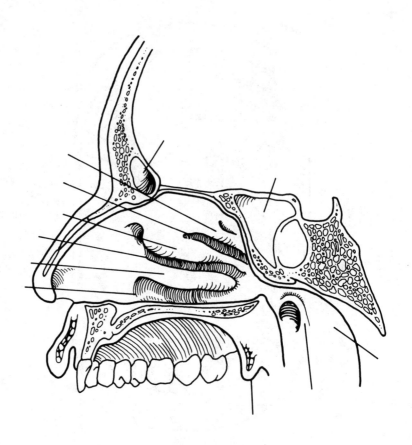

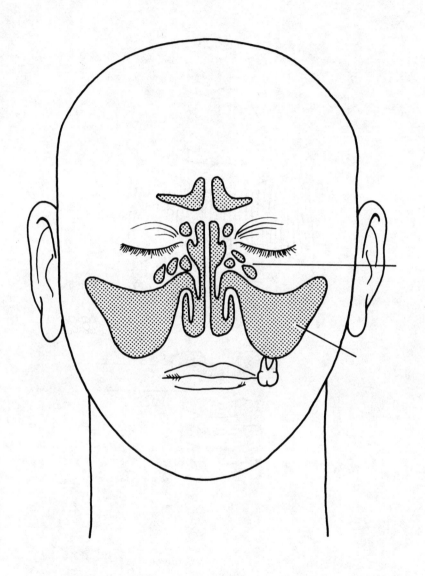

217

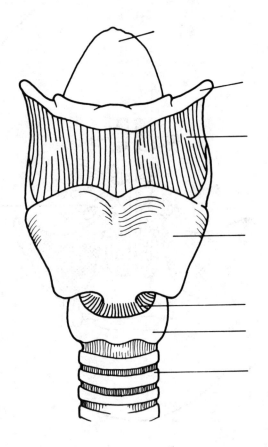

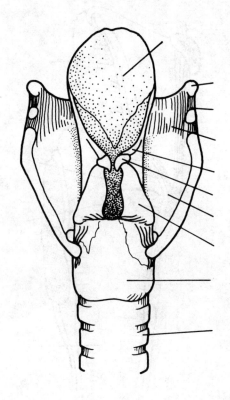

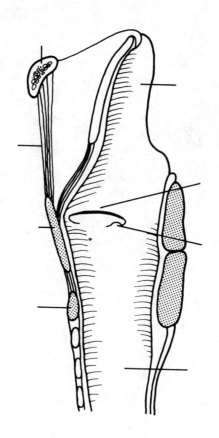

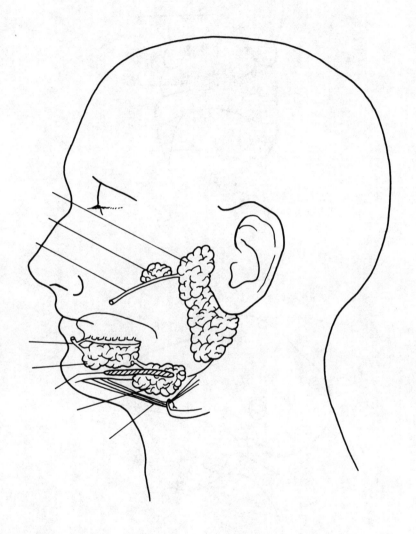

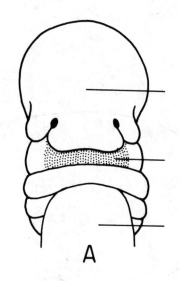

A

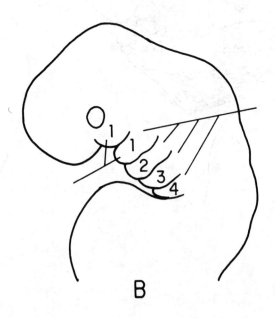

B

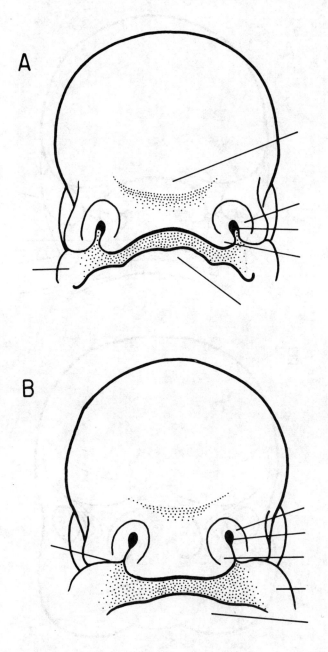

A

B

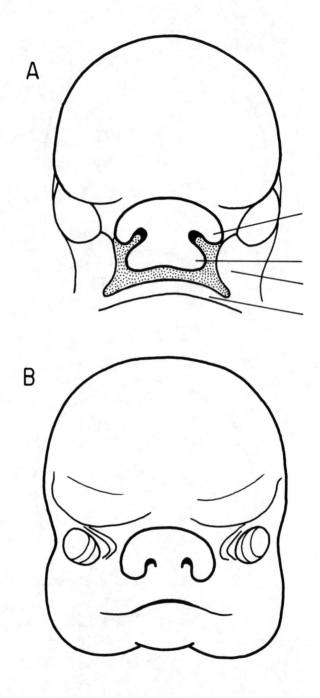

A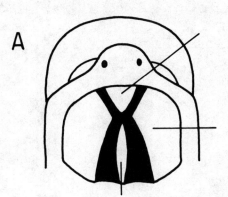

B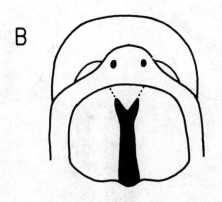

C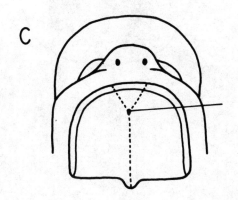

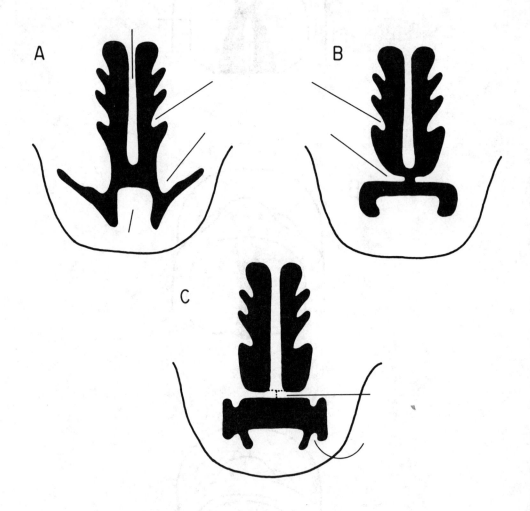

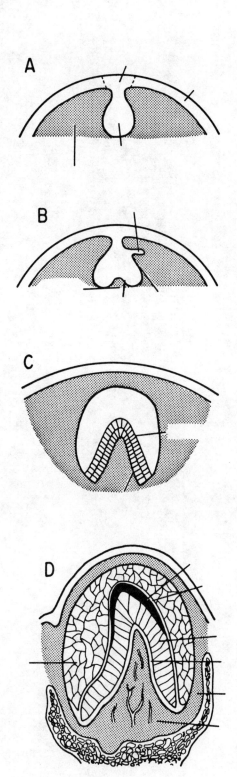

INDEX

KALAMAZOO VALLEY
COMMUNITY COLLEGE

Presented By

Theresa Hollowell

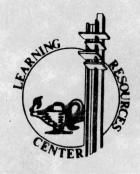